AF541429

URBANISATION, SLUMS AND ENVIRONMENTAL HEALTH

URBANISATION, SLUMS AND ENVIRONMENTAL HEALTH

N.A. Adinarayanappa

ANMOL PUBLICATIONS PVT. LTD.
NEW DELHI - 110 002 (INDIA)

ANMOL PUBLICATIONS PVT. LTD.
H.O.: 4374/4B, Ansari Road, Daryaganj,
New Delhi-110 002 (India)
Ph.: 23278000, 23261597
B.O.: No. 1015, Ist Main Road, BSK IIIrd Stage
IIIrd Phase, IIIrd Block,
Bangalore - 560 085 (India)
Visit us at: www.anmolpublications.com

Urbanisation, Slums and Environmental Health

ISBN 978-81-261-3662-9

PRINTED IN INDIA

Printed at Mehra Offset Press, Delhi.

CONTENTS

CONTENTS

PREFACE

The present book is exclusively based on the findings of my doctoral research entitled, "Slums, Urban Environment and Health – A Sociological study of Bangalore city". An attempt has been made here to examine the nature of interconnection and the process of interaction across Urbanisation, proliferation of slums and environmental degradation. Though Urbanisation has received the maximum attention of environmental scientists and town planners, indeed very few attempts have been made to examine the problems of Urbanisation in the context of the inter-linkages that seem to exist across Urbanisation, slums and environmental degradation.

During the course of my M.Phil work, I realized the need for looking at slums from the view point of environmental health. Most of the studies on slums have stopped at best at analyzing the social problems like moral degradation, urban crime, commercial sex, family disorganisation, personality disorganisation, alcoholism, beggary to mention, but a few. So much so, it may be appropriate to call these studies as social pathological studies. No doubt, these studies have thrown lot of light on the causes, course and consequences of social problems. Rich research out put brought out by these studies has been incorporated in formulating and designing a number of policies and programmes for urban development. It is a pity that in almost all these studies the environmental impact of these social problems and slums in particular has remained the least explored aspect of sociological studies.

Given the serious concern with which environment is looked upon at the present juncture, the present study takes departure from the above and seeks to assess the impact of slums on environment and naturally acquires a phenomenal significance and importance. Hence, an attempt has been made here to highlight the environmental degradation and its consequences on urban environment and health.

There is an enormous scope for further studies in this field and a lot more interesting facts can emerge which would help to frame policies and plans for betterment of the society by the urban town-planners, environmental activists, social scientists and government to mention a few.

Large number of persons has helped me in completing this work. First and foremost, I shall remain deeply indebted to my guide Dr. Y. Narayana Chetty, Professor and Chairman, Department of Sociology, Bangalore University, for his continuous help, support and guidance without which the book would not have been completed. I also remain grateful to my teaching staff of the Department of Sociology, Dr. G. Sivaramakrishnan, Dr. R. Venkatasubbaiah, Dr. C. Somashekar, Dr. R. Rajesh, and Dr. B. Samatha Deshmane, for their moral support. My heartfelt thanks to Dr. C.G. Lakshmipathi, N.S.S. co-ordinator, Bangalore University.

I am also deeply indebted to my parents, Sri. Adeppa and Rathnamma, my father-in-law, Sri. P.V. Prakash, my wife Smt. Veenarani.P, my brother Sri. N. A. Rangappa and family and my daughter Kum. N. A. Hamsa Shree for their continuous support.

I would also like to extend my gratitude to Prof. Jogan Shankar, professor and Chairman of the Department of Sociology and Dr. Gurulingaiah, Mangalore University, Prof. S. L. Hiremath, Department of Sociology, Gulbarga University, Dr. C. Somashekarappa, Chairman, the Department of Sociology, Dharwad University, prof. Panchaksharaiah, Dr. Ramegowda and Dr. Chandrashekar, Kuvempu University, Shimoga and J.M. Mallikarjunaiah, principal, K.L.E's Law College, Bangalore, Dr. Sudha Seetharam, Government Arts College, Bangalore and principal Sri. Kumaraswamy and colleagues of Basaveshwara Degree College, Vijayanagar, Bangalore.

I am thankful to Prof. T.H. Eranna, Joint Director, Collegiate Education, Bangalore region, Bangalore and family, V. Sambaji Rao, Assistant Director, Collegiate Education, Bangalore region, Bangalore, Dr. Rajashekar Reddy, Assistant Director, Collegiate Education, Bangalore region, Bangalore.

I also thank Sri. Uday Kumar S. Kollimath, Marketing Specialist, Jala Samvardhane Yojana Sangha. My heartfelt gratitude to Sri. J.L. Kumar, Managing Director and Sri. V. Srinivasa Murthy, Branch Manger(South), Anmol Publications Pvt. Ltd, New Delhi for their generous help to bring out this book at the earliest possible.

Dr. N. A. Adinarayanappa

ACRONYMS

• ACs	:	Air Coolers
• ARI	:	Acute Respiratory Infection
• ARI	:	Acute Respiratory Infections.
• ATB	:	Association for Tropical Biology
• ATREE	:	Ashoka Trust for Research in Ecology and the Environment
• BMIC	:	Bangalore-Mysore Infrastructure Corridor
• BUA	:	Bangalore Urban Agglomeration.
• BWSSB	:	Bangalore Water Supply and Sewerage Board
• Cb	:	Cobalt
• CBOs	:	Community Based Organisations
• Cd	:	Cadmium.
• CEERA	:	Centre for Environmental Law, Education, Research and Advocacy
• CFE	:	Consent for Establishment
• CFO	:	Consent for Operation
• CLP	:	China Light and Power
• CMC	:	City Municipal Corporation.
• CO	:	Carbon Monoxide
• CPCB	:	Central Pollution Control Board.
• Cr	:	Chromium.
• CRT	:	Cathode Ray Tube

• Cu	:	Copper
• DDS		Deccan Development Society
• ECAs	:	Export Credit Agencies
• EIA	:	Environment Impact Assessment
• EMPRI	:	Environmental Management and Policy Research Institute
• EPA	:	Environmental Protection Agency.
• ESG	:	Environment Support Group
• GOI	:	Government of India.
• GW	:	Ground Water
• HC	:	High Court
• HC	:	Hydro Carbons
• IPP Station	:	Indraprastha Power Station.
• KSPCB	:	Karnataka State Pollution Control Board
• LSGs	:	Local Self Governments
• Ltd.	:	Limited
• M. Corp	:	Municipal Corporation.
• mg/m_3	:	Milligram, Meter Cube
• MOU	:	Memorandum of Understanding
• MPCL	:	Murdeshwar Power Corporation Ltd.
• MW	:	Mega Watts
• MW	:	Molecular Weight
• NEC	:	Foundation for Natural Exploration and Environmental Conservation
• NGOs	:	Non-governmental Organisations.
• Ni	:	Nickel
• NLSIU	:	National Law School of India University

• NO	:	Nitrogen Oxide
• NOx	:	Nitrus Oxide
• O_3	:	Ozone
• OGs	:	Out Growths
• PAHs	:	Poly-aromatic hydrocarbons.
• Pb	:	Lead.
• PM	:	Particulate mater.
• PPAs	:	Power Purchase Agreements
• PVC	:	Poly Venyl Chloride
• RBI	:	Reserve Bank of India
• REIA	:	Rapid Environment Impact Assessment
• RPM	:	Repairable Particulate Mater
• SACON	:	Salim Ali Centre for Ornithology and Natural History
• SANA	:	South Asia North America Environmental Justice
• SC	:	Supreme Court
• So_2	:	Sulphur Dioxide
• Sox	:	Sulphur Oxide
• TERI	:	Tata Energy Research Institute
• TMC	:	Town Municipal Corporation.
• TP	:	Taluk Panchayath.
• TRI	:	Toxic Release Inventory
• TSP	:	Total Suspended Particulate.
• UK	:	United Kingdom
• UNESCAP	:	United Nations Economic and Social Commission For Asia Pacific
• US	:	United States.
• USA	:	United States of America

• UTs	:	Union Territories
• WHO	:	World Health Organisation.
• WT	:	Water Table
• Zn	:	Zinc.

CHAPTER I

INTRODUCTION

An attempt has been made here to examine the nature of interconnection and the process of interaction across Urbanisation, proliferation of slums and the environmental degradation. The phenomenon of environmental degradation in the form of pollution of air, water, soil and noise primarily due to enormous increase in vehicular traffic, discharge of effluents by industrial units and generation of unlimited unwieldy solid waste, not to speak of rapid depletion of resources due to rapid growth of population in general and urban population in particular. It has received the maximum attention of environmental scientists, town planners. These developments agitated the mind of environmental activists and socially sensitive sociologists. Indeed very few attempts have been made to examine these problems in the context of the inter-linkages that seem to exist across Urbanisation, slums and environmental degradation.

Conventionally slums, as social disorganisations have received the maximum attention of urban sociologists. Most of these studies have stopped at best at analysing the social problems like moral degradation, urban crime, commercial sex, family disorganisation, personality disorganisation, alcoholism, beggary to mention, but a few. So much so, it may be appropriate to call these studies as social pathological studies. No doubt, these studies have thrown lot of light on the causes, course and consequences of social problems. Rich research out put brought out by these studies has been incorporated in formulating and designing a number of policies and programmes for urban development. It is a pity that in almost all these studies the environmental impact of these social problems and slums in particular has remained the least explored aspect of sociological studies. Given the serious concern with which environment is looked upon at the present juncture. The present study naturally acquires a phenomenal significance and importance.

One of the inevitable and almost unavoidable social consequences of Urbanisation and industrialisation has been the unabated proliferation of slums accompanied by environmental degradation among much else. Slums created in this way have come to pose many serious problems to urban communities. Social problems of industrial cities have received the maximum and serious attention of sociologists and social anthropologists. Slums and the environmental degradation is one such serious problem which has so far received hardly any serious attention of sociologists. One of the causes of growth of slums as has been noted rather repeatedly is the rural-urban migration. Lack of employment opportunities, crop failures, famines, floods and other natural calamities associated with farming and allied occupations in rural areas have forced rural population to move over to towns and cities. Without necessary skills, knowledge and training required to carry out highly specialised technical jobs that are available in cities most rural migrants tend to find wide-variety of casual jobs in the informal and unorganised sectors like building construction, petty-trade and business, domestic service, vendors, hawkers and a host of other low-paid menial and manual activities. Inevitably these people find shelter wherever they find vacant unclaimed lands however inhospitable and unhygienic they may be for a stable and sustainable living.

Environmental changes and implications in India:

From the view point of the study of environmental changes and their impact on the study involves an examination of India, one of the world's largest and most populous countries. It is essentially an examination of a microcosm of the earth. Its populace encompasses the entire range of the income and education spectra, its culture consists of diverse religions, languages, and social systems, and its geography is a sample of almost every terrestrial climatic zone of the planet. It is this variation that makes India's environment so interesting. India holds the dubious honour of suffering from poverty-induced environmental degradation. It is a tricky task to understand the complexities behind the state of India's environment. Furthermore, these problems are most likely to become complicated in the years to come, as India remains one of the fastest growing countries in the world, in terms of population as well as economy. To gain an understanding of what is really going on within India and its environment; one needs to look at a whole gamut of socio-economic and bio-physical parameters.

Poverty, particularly in the form of inadequate nutrition, has presented a persistent problem for India. Although not a necessary outcome of a growing population, it often comes about when the agricultural and economic engines of a region are not able to keep up with food demand, and the aggregate production of the country is not being adequately distributed.

The second aspect of population of concern is that of consumption. Even at a constant per capita consumption rate, the sheer increase in numbers will translate to a massive increase in the burden on India. And as the large masses continue their struggle of maintaining even this modest level of subsistence, they act in ways that degrade the environment, particularly in the form of damage to their soil and drinking water supplies.

However, besides the environmental impacts from subsistence consumption, continued economic growth has translated to a more than doubling in per capita net national product between 1950 and 1990 What this means is that the average person may be demanding substantially more natural resources, generating substantially more pollution, and discarding substantially more waste. And since economic theory states that as income increases, people spend a smaller portion of their income on food, and more on other types of goods (like automobiles and appliances), this might result in the form of worst environmental damage. As we will see in the subsequent chapters, the increase in aggregate consumption has indeed had its impacts on air pollution, water pollution, land degradation and a host of other negative environmental changes.

'Slum population and environmental changes is the core of the thesis', what has sociology to do with environment and environmental studies and *vise-versa* has been a matter of great deal of discussion. Discovered at a time when the field of environmental studies has been dominated by physical and natural sciences, sociologists and social anthropologists came to evince some interest on the subject though belatedly. Two issues received the attention of the sociologists. They are:

1. The causes and consequences of environmental changes and degradation of environment in societies.
2. The role environmental politics can play to curb environmental degradation.

The Classical social theories of Karl Marx, Weber and Durkheim don't seem to take a serious note of environmental issues. Weber's work shows the least engagement with the natural world. Even Marx and Durkheim, who saw the relations between human societies and the natural world as central to historical change, did not pay much attention to the impact of economic and demographic processes on ecosystems. (Indira Munshi, 254, 2000).

However, scholars like Ted Benton argue that there is much in the corpus of Marxian historical materialism which is compatible with an ecological perspective. (Benton, 1989:63)

Limited legacy though in social theory that it does not have adequate conceptual frame work to understand the complex interaction between society and environment, sociologist's failure to recognize the negative impact that Industrialisation and Urbanisation has produced on environment could be one reason responsible for the neglect of environmental issues or concern in the main stream of sociological theory. It is hardly surprising that ecological variables are hardly incorporated in sociological analysis. However, in recent times, environmental concerns both the nature of environmental degradation and the emergence of environmental movements has been articulated in sociological research.

Among the pioneers who showed the great interest and sensitivity to their relationship between humans and their environment was Patrick Geddes, the founder of Sociology Department at Bombay University. Urbanisation and Industrialisation accompanied by profound technological changes have altered the relationship of man, animal and nature. Geddes devoted much of his time and energy to the task of planning the urban environment with a view to preserving the best historical traditions. He emphasised the need for the involvement of the people in management of environmental resources. The large number of reports which he prepared on Indian cities bear testimony to his commitment to improve the urban environment in order to enhance the quality of life of people. Radha Kamal Mukherjee, carried on Geddes' legacy with zeal. (Anthony Giddens; Ulrich Beck; Clause Offe; Jargon; Habermas and others have addressed themselves environmental issues. For a critical review of their contribution see "Environment" in sociological theory - Indira Munshi from pages, 256, to 259, 2000).

Delhi-based Centre for Science and Environment brought out two reports on the state of India's environment in the year 1982 and 1985. These reports throw a lot of light on factors responsible for deterioration of environmental quality. Media particularly the print media through newspapers and journals have been reporting on a variety of issues related to environmental degradation over a decade or so. Environmental activities consistently carried on major battles against the projects initiated by the government. Social activist groups have organised down to earth struggle at local and national levels against, the increasing control over natural resources by vested-interests including the state to the determinant of local communities. Ramachandra Guha made a pioneering effort in conducting studies of village ecosystems. Centre for Appropriate Science and Technology for Rural Areas setup at the Indian Institute of Sciences in Bangalore has made a note worthy work under the leadership of A. K. N. Reddy, Professor of Chemistry. The centre carried out a number of studies. The out put turned out by these studies have been immensely useful in designing environmentally sound development projects. He has been advocating a development strategy which has come to be known as 'eco-development'. The main objective of this development strategy is to provide for the satisfaction of basic needs of the poor; endogenous self-reliance in terms of using local raw materials and through social participation and control over resources and harmony with the environment. (Guha, 1997; 347)

Several studies have focused on the social and environmental consequences of colonial state intervention, its effect on the indigenous social, cultural institutions and practices of resource management; and social protests over control of resources (See Guha 1989; Rangarajan,1996; Arnold and Guha, 1994; Munshi, 1993; Whitcombe, 1972; Sengupta, 1980; Tucker, 1979; Grove, 1995).

Depletion of natural resources in the contemporary context, the changed used and management of these resources and their effect on local communities, and the need for an alternative system of resource management have been the subjects of many studies conducted by social scientist in general (See Jodha, 1986; Chopra *et al.*, 1989; Fernandes and Menon, 1987; Nadkarni, 1989; Agarwal, 1986). There has been some discussion on gender and environment and on the notion of eco-feminism in recent times (Shiva, 1988; Agarwal, 1991, 1997; Venkateshwaran, 1995).

Displacement, marginalisation and deterioration of the quality of life of large sections of the population, the tribals, nomadic communities, craftsmen, the urban and the rural poor and women, as a result of the economic policies of the government have concerned both social scientists and activists alike. The aim is to work out an alternative framework of development which would combine sustainability with equality and social justice. It can hardly be overstated that everywhere in the developing countries, as in India, protests and struggles by rural and urban communities for control, access and management of natural resources upon which their lives and livelihood depend, are taking place and gaining worldwide recognition. Friedman and Rangan call it 'Environmental action' (1993:4).

Contemporary ecological movements, especially the Chipko movement and the Narmada Bachao Andolan, as well as conflicts over natural resources like water, forest and fisheries have recently found a place in social science research in India (Shiva, 1991; Gadgil and Guha, 1996; Baviskar, 1995; Kurien, 1993; Berreman, 1989; Jai, 1984; Omvedt, 1987). Conflicts/struggles over forest, water, fish, land, pasture and village commons being widespread all over the country, many studies on these aspects are needed; it is also a fact that there is a tradition of study of social movements in sociology. (Indira Munshi, *'Environment' in Sociological Theory*. Sociological Bulletin, 49 (2), Sep.2000)

Key Concepts: A Discussion

Health:

Given lot of myths surrounding our conception of health, different people tend to look at health in different ways. One of the ways in which it has been defined is in terms of absence of symptoms of disease. This is taken as a sign of good health. Fact of the matter however is not as simple as this could imply. Absence of symptoms of disease cannot be regarded as sign of good health because symptoms take a fairly long time before they show up and that health specialists could differ from one another in reading and interpreting the exact meaning of the symptoms. The extent to which symptoms show up depends however upon such factors as the type of ailment, age, sex, family background of the patient to mention but few factors. Alternately and increasingly in terms of Behavioural sciences, health is defined, "as a person's capacity to carry out one's day-to-day activities with a certain amount of confidence, efficiency and competency". Ideally, health refers to the social, psychological, physical, cultural and economic well-being of a person. At the outset one may wonder as to what exactly Sociology has to do with health. During the last two decades or so, there has been a growing interest in the preventive possibilities of relationship between peoples' health and features of social and economic environment in which people live. Environmental changes that followed have been absolutely beyond control of individuals.

There is considerable body of empirical evidence to show that adverse work environment and low occupational status are linked with metabolic disturbances which are not explained by obesity, smoking, alcohol consumption and/or exercise pattern. Socio-economic differences in health conditions were a reflection of differences in the circumstances in which people live and work. These differences are the inevitable part of the lot of people and tend to impinge upon and affect the health of people. Another way of defining health is that health is a state of complete physical, mental and social well-being and not merely absence of disease or infirmity (WHO, 1946). Much of discussion on health almost exclusively deals with diseases and causes. Illness is a devalued process that impairs the functioning or appearance of a person and may ultimately lead to death. Definition of health given by WHO emphasizes on the social, physical and mental well-being of a person. Among other things this reflects a concern with total personality of human and the person as a member of human groups – an entity certainly not limited to the body of that person. Other components of an individual for example blood, body, soul, spirit, shadow and name, etc. are defined differently in one culture and another.

Disease, illness then, may involve a temporary or permanent impairment in the functioning of any single component or of the relationship between components making up an individual. Any impairment, leads to a decrease in a person's ability to function efficiently in day-to-day situation. For example, among the Ashanthi of West Africa, a congenital birthmark which leads to no discomfort or danger of death can be considered a sufficiently severe fault to disqualify a man from the office of chief. In many cultures theories of disease will include explanations of congenital defects or imperfections, and the distinction between these and other illness may become relevant for further analysis (Polgar, 1963).

Diagnosis, therapy and prophylaxis are three basic elements of all medical systems. The causes of the disease are explained by two concepts

1. Notions of singular causation and, 2. Multi-causal conceptions of disease.

The former was much in practice during the last decades of 19th century and the early part of the 20th century. For ex.: the Western medicine was heavily dominated by the notion that most diseases are a result of infection caused by microorganisms. The emergence of the "doctrine of specific etiology of disease", Dubos [(1959) 1961, p.90] as the dominant idea in medicine is related to the mechanistic world view prevalent in the late 19th century.

In contemporary practice of clinical medicine, inadequate care often received by patients might unfortunately aggravate disability for which no specific etiology can be identified. Inefficiency, neglect whether intended or unintended on the part of medical practitioners might lead to unanticipated consequences sometimes leading to permanent disability or death. This could be an example of social organisation of medical case.

The recent theoretical developments marked a shift from the doctrine of specific etiology to a comprehensive medical care and psychosomatic medicine and psychotherapies. There has been a growing realisation in medical community of the fact that illness is an outcome of interaction of many factors and correspondingly favours treatment of patients more as total organism in a complex setting. One of the foremost modern exponents of this view is the epidemiologist John Gordon, who has shown the interplay of the host, the agent, and the (physical, biological and social) environment in the spread of a good number of both infectious and non-infectious diseases. Although writers in the psychosomatic tradition of medicine often use concepts like 'stress' or 'conflict' as if they were specific causes of illness, the emphasis in this school of thought is on the patient's physical and mental well-being, and consideration is often given to his social milieu as well (King, 1963). Comprehensive medical care is thus, more than a movement to improve the institutional means by which patients and sometimes families are medically supervised.

The multi-causal conceptions of disease are neither new in the Western medical tradition nor unique to it. One main theme in the Hippocratic writings is that disease is to be traced to an imbalance between the person and his external environment; much emphasis is also given to the relationships among different environmental factors, such as exercise and diet, and to the connections between disturbances in an organ and the whole body. In non-western societies as well there are many multi-causal ideas about disease.

In urban as well as non-urban societies, the search for the transgression of the patient himself or the malevolent action of another being (human or supernatural) is a major element of the diagnostic process. If disease is seen as an individual's departure from perfectly well-meshed social or physiological performance, health, by contrast, becomes an asymptote – an ideal that can be approached but never attained in actuality. In the WHO definition, the expression "complete physical, mental and social well-being" [emphasis added] echoes this type of conception. (Sigerist, 1951-1956, vol.2, pp.317 ff; Dubos, 1959, 1961, pp.117)

In recent times, the de-institutionalised approach is increasingly gaining acceptance as the most appropriate mode of treatment. In the present modern medical practice, in terms of actual health Behaviour in urban societies, open-ended conceptions are more likely to be put into practice in national parks, beauty parlours, bathrooms, or athletic studios than in the offices of doctors or psychologists. Physicians may recommend vacations, walks in the 'fresh-air', or other types of exercises, but this is usually prescribed for incipient illness or problems of overweight rather than promoting health as such. In non-Western societies one may find practices aimed at increasing supernatural power, physical strength, prosperity, wisdom, virility, or femininity, which are conceptually and Behaviourally integrated which actions to prevent or cure disease. In industrialised societies however, increased specialisation results in the separation of medical institutions from the religious, esthetic, recreational and economic spheres. Thus, the doctrine of specific etiology of disease become the dominant view and health promotion through such customs as taking cold showers, swallowing vitamin pills to "pep you up", giving laxatives routinely to children, taking walks and the like is seldom transmitted as part of the professional medical system but rather is passed thorough relatives, friends, or the mass media. The relationship between people and their environment becomes the central arena of medical profession.

Development of a full blown disease is encouraged by the kind of life experiences that wrench the person from the accustomed interpersonal environment that exposes him to the social stress of isolation and probably to a corresponding degradation or disarray the self-image of a person. Bulk of illness notably including mental illness is found among the separated, divorced, widowed and single population. Such persons allege to be highly vulnerable to high health risks in comparison to the persons who live in intact socially, psychologically cohesive family units. Since, slum is a social disorganisation the consequences of disintegration of social institutions over there are reflected in high health risk behaviours of slum dwellers. Slums also represent the most disadvantaged sectors of population. Diseases are rampant not only due to the obvious defects of nutrition, housing, preventive medical care, etc, but, also it is a syndrome of social and psychological insufficiency. This syndrome may be visualised in terms of generalised inferiority feelings, a defect in the self image, generalised incompetence–defect in the trained capacity to function in the rewarded social roles. Therefore, if we wish to understand distribution of ill health in population we must pay attention not only to the conventional hazards of physical environment and microorganisms but also to the social relations and psychological characteristics that permeates life history of the people. Sociology emphasizes man's wholeness, his/her simultaneous existence as biological, psychological and social creature. Sociological thinking on health thus, marks a point of departure. The so called physical approach to illness and treatment to which people are very much accustomed to is not only one sided but also has serious unintended side effects.

Current research and theory is concerned with the influence of mental state on the illness of the physical body. Physical aspects of disease - the organic manifestations which we have come to regard as the disease itself may in fact represent a comparatively late stage in the underlying dysfunction. Treating illness by means of conventional methods like drugs, surgery, radiation amounts to scratching the surface of the problem. Physical interventions may at best attend to the symptoms of basic affliction rather than to the real causes. Holistic approach to health therefore includes careful consideration of factors emanating from socio-economic environment.

It has become well known that a person's behaviour and disturbed mental state relate to his/her chances of becoming ill. Sociology as a science of human behaviour tells us that a person's state of mind depends upon and determined by his/her social relations with others. Slum as a social disorganisation, social relations have been the casualties. We believe the slum populations are increasingly vulnerable to and might actually suffer from serious psycho-somatic disorders let alone other disorders. An attempt is made in the present study to study the nature of diseases, distribution of diseases, causes and consequences of diseases among slum population and the social consequences of such diseases and high health risk behaviour of slum population on a wider society – the urban living environment.

Environment

The concept of environment refers to all sorts of surroundings and includes material, social and spiritual conditions of living beings. When we consider it as a physical entity, environmental problems are consequences of human interventions. The human causation of environmental problems may be clarified by the difference between natural and environmental catastrophes. Former being a dramatic change of the environment caused by natural process without human interventions and the latter changes are caused primarily by human interventions. The three broad categories of environmental problems are exhaustion, pollution and disturbance.

Exhaustion refers to the depletion of natural resources both renewable and non-renewable. Minerals and fossil fuels are non- renewable resources. Their stocks are fixed. Different forms of pollution of air, water and soil, disturbances of ecosystems and damage to the scenic beauty of landscapes are among the negative impacts associated with extraction of minerals and fossil fuels. The over use of non-renewable materials often leads to exhaustion and they may no longer be available in future.

Renewable resources are those which include both abiotic components like soil and water and biotic components like plants and animals. Their renewal takes place as a completely natural process or be stimulated by human interventions. These may exhaust directly when the use of resource exceeds its reproduction or indirectly when the conditions for reproduction are disturbed or when existing stocks are destroyed or made unusable.

Used materials whether or not transformed into solid, fluid or gaseous waste, sooner or later return into the environment. In case of exhaustion the environment is used as a storehouse which could get depleted. Pollution can be defined as the release of harmful substances into the environment. Besides pollution, there are other environmental effects of human Behaviour which are experienced as annoying or risky ex: noise, radiation and heat. These experiences are termed as 'Environmental stresses'.

Forms of environmental pollution may be divided into flux-type and sink-type pollution. Well known forms of flux-type pollution are air pollution and surface water pollution. This can only be reduced by reducing the emission of pollutants into streams. In recent decades several countries have been successful in reducing the concentration of sulphur dioxide in the air and of heavy metals in surface waters.

Reduction of concentrations of substances in air and water does not end the accumulation of these substances at fixed places like soils and river beds. This process of accumulation is called sink-type pollution. Several contemporary environmental problems such as the pollution of soils, river beds and ground water wells as well as acidification and the enhanced green house effect are cases of sink-type pollution.

Environmental problems do not only originate in taking too much out of it or dumping too much into it but also in the disruption by human activities of a relationship which occur and processes which take place between different elements both abiotic and biotic of the environment. This is referred to as 'Environmental disturbance'.

It is impossible to prevent all environmental problems. Human beings cannot live without changing their environment. Human beings have to change their environment to protect themselves against climatic influences like high or low temperatures, precipitation, sunshine, wind and floods and against poisonous plants and dangerous animals. They also have to provide themselves with food, water, materials and heat. It is unavoidable that these types of human changes in the environment are sometimes interpreted as problematic.

However, there are three major factors which contribute to the growing impact of human Behaviour on the physical environment: increasing numbers of people and the growing quantity and changing quality of human use of the environment.

- Increasing numbers of people
- Growing quantity of human use of the environment
- Changing quality of human use of the environment

The more the people are living together, the more likely human influence on the environment will be experienced as problematic. In recent decades, in wealthy western countries all kinds of environmentally degrading activities have been increased much more than the sheer numbers of human beings. Population growth is a major cause of increasing environmental stress.

Not only the growing numbers of people but also the growth of their per capita use of environmental resources contributes to contemporary environmental problems. In general, economic growth leads to a larger utilisation of natural resources. There is often a strong correlation between economic growth and growth of energy use and hence, economic growth together with population growth, has often been considered as a major cause of environmental problems. Both private and public activities do cause environmental problems.

The production of economic goods and services may be associated with widely different quantities of materials used and pollutants emitted. According to Barry Commoner there is striking evidence that production of most basic needs - food, clothing, and housing - consumed 40 to 50 *per cent* of resources. Increase in population led to changes in the manner in which we use resources. The kind of goods produced to meet these needs have changed drastically. New production technologies have displaced old ones. Soap powder has been displaced by synthetic detergents; natural fibres (cotton and wool) have been displaced by synthetic ones; steel and lumber have been displaced by aluminum, plastics, and concrete; railroad freight has been displaced by truck freight; returnable bottles have been displaced by non-returnable ones. On the road, the low-powered automobile engines of the 1920's and 1930's have been displaced by high-powered ones. On the farm, while per capita production has remained constant, the amount of harvested acreage has decreased; in effect, fertiliser has displaced land". (Commoner, 1971, pp.141-142)

This qualitative aspect is not only dependent on technological developments but also on organisational or managerial developments. Whether production processes or products are more or less exhausting or polluting the environment is not only determined by technology but also by the way industrial production is organised.

The quality of human-induced change of the environment does not always develop in a negative way. Modernisation in production technologies in recent years have resulted in reduction of negative environmental effects of these processes and products. The term 'Ecological modernisation' has been introduced to indicate this development (Huber, 1982).

Environmental issues are socially determined. Why do activities continue largely unchecked even after it has become clear that they are harmful to the environment? There are apparently forces at work in our society which ensure that activities which are extremely damaging to that society nevertheless continue to take place. Environmental problems arise because the detrimental effects of a particular intervention. This invariably involves different sections of society who would get benefits from that intervention. In other words, there are always groups in society which have a vested interest in some activities beneficial to them no matter how harmful to others. Vested-interests play a decisive role in the origin of environmental problems.

The separation of advantages and disadvantages is often spatial. Much of the pollution of air, rivers and seas causes problems which go beyond the boundaries of a single nation. For example, when nuclear power plants are planned, there are noticeable preferences for locations near the border; not only does the river provide cooling water, but waste water flows out of the country. The processing of household refuse, whether by dumping or incineration, is usually concentrated in a particular locality. The local communities bear the brunt of the disadvantages, while the benefits, in the form of cheap and simple disposal of refuse, go to households elsewhere in the country. The addition of phosphates to fertilizer and copper to pig feeds means that these substances enter the soil in a non-concentrated form and cannot be reclaimed. If continued, this practice is expected to cause enormous problems for future generations.

Air and noise pollution maybe treated as individual advantages over collective disadvantages as anyone responsible for the emission of harmful gases through the chimney or in the form of exhaust fumes is polluting everyone's environment. The contribution of single motorist to air pollution is relatively small, as is the noise pollution produced by a single automobile. But the benefit provided by that automobile are reserved exclusively for the motorist himself. In all such cases, where the detrimental effects on the environment are more or less immediate, the burdens to the 'perpetrator' are always smaller than the advantages he enjoys, precisely because the burdens are passed on to society as a whole.

The conservation of environment seldom benefits only the individual; it is almost always to the good of the entire society. Environmental components all serve one or more functions in society. The sociological concept of function stands for an objectively observable consequence or effect of human activity. An environmental function is an effect or result of circumstances in the environment which is of significance for society. In most cases this means the practical value of certain environmental components, such as clean air to breathe, natural resources to exploit, or simply scenic beauty to enjoy. In an economic sense each of the various functions of he environment for society can be considered a commodity or a 'good' for which there is demand and supply. Although there may be considerable differences between these environmental goods, they are almost always public or collective goods.

Environmental damage reduces the availability of environmental functions, and thus the availability of collective goods. The crux of the problem is how individuals can be motivated to cause least harm to the environment. (*Society and Its Environment- An Introduction,* by Egbert Tellegen and Maarten Wolsink, pp. No. 6-21 & 83-90, University of Amsterdam, The Netherlands, 1994)

Urbanisation

In the past two decades the world's urban population has increased by about a billion from 1.35 to 2.28 billion. The bulk of this increase has been (about 60 per cent) in Asia and most of it in the South Asian countries. As per the estimates, urban population is close to 400 million in South Asia. This will increase to 800 million in 20 years. In most South Asian cities, urban infrastructure built slowly over several decades, is already under severe strain with continuous migration from rural areas. Rural migrants in search of better living conditions in urban areas, remain below the acceptable threshold even though urban living conditions have improved over in the last 50 years since independence. The cities will find it extremely difficult to cope with demands for civic services and basic infrastructure. Low income groups will create slums.

The spatial context of Urbanisation should also be considered with reference to the process of formation of metropolitan regions and urbanised areas. The conditions–

social, economic, technological, demographic, required for generating and consolidating forces of Urbanisation and modernisation would depend not only on the population size of the urban Centre, but also on the functional character, and growth and history of the urban community. For instance, irrespective of the size of the population, the state capital would serve as a powerful nucleus for generation and transmission of the forces of urbanism and transformation of the life of the surrounding region. Unplanned growth of cities would, overtime, become Centres of squalor, squatter settlements, and slum, irregular and haphazard human settlements. Needless to add that, the cumulative effect is urban environmental degradation and destruction of the life on earth.

The correlation between industrialisation and Urbanisation has been extensively investigated. Studies have shown that there could be Urbanisation without industrialisation such Urbanisation when happens the social character of Urbanisation would remain unchanged. They become what are called 'Urban villages'. Urban villages are environmentally unsound. The pace of Urbanisation in the underdeveloped countries much more closely depends on the pace of industrialisation than in the highly industrialised areas.

M.S.A Rao found that urban employment and development of trade and commerce have not only led to a greater differentiation of occupational roles than that caused by commercialisation of agriculture, but have also resulted in different combinations of occupations on the one hand and occupational mobility on the other. S.N. Agarwal (1970) conducted a demographic study of six urbanising villages in the Union Territory of Delhi. He covered aspects like households, heads of households, village population, marriage and divorce, widowhood, separation and remarriage, fertility control, infant and child mortality, birth and death rates. Except providing statistical details, he has not tried to analyze how these can be related to urban influence *vice-versa.*

From the foregoing appraisal of studies it is obvious that the various demographic elements cannot be studied in isolation. These are the products of multi-linked processes and these, in turn, serve as factors contributing to the changes in other aspects including environmental changes.

Population

Whether population is the cause of poverty or poverty is the cause of over population has been the most persistent source of raging controversy and confusion one thing seems certain from the point of view of environment; namely, that rapid growth of population resulted almost inevitably in environmental degradation which in turn accentuated poverty. Poverty has innumerable forms and the form in which it has manifested most is maldistribution of environmental resources, increasing level of malnutrition, inadequate nutrition and the increasing vulnerability of vast mass of population to disease, disability, starvation and even death. It could be argued that poverty is not necessarily an outcome of growing population although in the present circumstances it has something to do with that. It often comes about also due to declining levels of agricultural output particularly when coupled with equally declining levels of economic and industrial productivity. This results in as already pointed out in the maldistribution of the total output and also inadequate access to resources and opportunities to majority of population in a region. Analysing the relationship between untouchables and poverty is measured in terms of income and calories intake. It was found that the base number of food calories intake is daily 2,400 calories for rural population and 2,100 for urban population whereas, the calories requirement for India, based on lifestyle and climatic factors is 2,150 calories per day (UNDP, 1995). However, there has been a gradual increase in the calories intake from 2197 in 1984 to 2395 in

1992. The increase in calories intake is so slow and sporadic that it has made, if any, least difference in the quality life of general population. There is increasing evidence of the link between increase in poverty and sexually transmitted diseases (STDs) including HIV/AIDS. In Thailand, the AIDS NGO network expresses concern that economic crisis may further marginalize HIV/AIDS patients (Deepa Narayan, 2002, pp.117).

Attempts have seldom been made to look at health from the point of view of environment and vice versa in the context of Urbanisation. Over the last five decades remarkable increase in transportation and communication has occurred in the developing world in general and India in particular. One of the most significant and visible development has been the huge exodus of people from rural to urban areas. While this has reaped many benefits such as increased economic development and higher income it has also brought with it serious environmental problems. Among other things this has resulted in unabated proliferation of slums and increased environmental degradation with adverse health implication. A healthy population is seldom found in an unhealthy environment. Slums have been a subject mater of a number of sociological studies; most studies have attempted to look at slums as social disorganisation. These studies have brought out abundant of information regarding various aspects of social life of people in slums, conditions of living of slum dwellers in towns and cities have become highly risky. Cities have become hotter than surrounding country-sides and have significant problems with flooding not to speak of chaotic urban traffic, increased crime rate, housing shortage, to mention a few. Diseases often spread through densely populated and poor communities and slum population is a classic case in point. Given this significant correlation between environment Urbanisation and health attempt has been made to discuss some aspects of the lifestyles of slum population in the following chapters.

References

1. Dhadave, M.S. 1988: *Sociology of slum,* Archives Books, New Delhi-55.
2. Tellegen, Egbert and Martin Wolsink, 1994: *Society and Its Environment. An Introduction,* University of Amsterdam, the Netherlands. pp. 6-21 and 81-90
3. *Guha, Ramachandra* 1989; *Rangarajan,*1996; *Arnold and Guha,* 1994; *Munshi,* 1993; *Whitcombe,* 1972; *Sengupta,* 1980; Tucker, 1979; Grove, 1995).
4. Munshi Indira, 2000: *'Environment' in Sociological Theory. Sociological Bulletin,* September 2000, pp. 258-262, Mumbai,
5. Parental Control, *Delayed marriage and population policies (Reports)* 1965: World Population Conference, Belgrade.
6. Srinivas M.N, and M.S.S Rao, 1974: *A Survey of Research in Sociology and Social Anthropology Vol. I, A Project sponsored by the Indian Council of Social Science Research,* New Delhi, Popular Prakashan, Bombay.
7. *The United Nations Development Programme (UNDP) 1997: Human Development Report.*
8. William, P. Reidhead, Suchi Guptha, Deepthi Joshi. *Tata Energy Research Institute,* 1996: State of India's Environment (A Qualitative Analysis).

CHAPTER II
ENVIRONMENTAL POLLUTION IN URBAN CITIES

Environmental Pollution

In recent decades, urban-centres in less-industrialised countries in general and India in particular have experienced unprecedented growth, and mega cities with populations of 10 million or more people have emerged in many countries. In India alone there are four such cities, with three others expected to join the ranks in the next 20 years. Globally, many rapidly growing cities are being overwhelmed by environmental problems, particularly air pollution. Deterioration of air quality is a problem that is directly experienced by a majority of the 300 million urban Indians, who constitute 30 per cent of India's population.

Mega cities of India are no exception to the global pattern of deteriorating urban air quality. Indian cities are among the most polluted in the world, with concentrations of a number of air pollutants being well above level as recommended by the World Health Organisation. Given the magnitude of pollution it is yet to be recognised as public health issue. Scientific understanding of health risks from air pollution in Indian cities is poor. There is a paucity of scientific studies on the health effects of air pollution. The few that have been done show much cause for alarm, and it is apparent to scientists and lay people alike that the residents of India's mega cities face significant risks to their health from exposure to air pollutants.

The dearth of data exists across the entire causal chain of risk assessment, from sources of pollution to atmospheric concentrations to human exposures and their health effects. Hardly anything is known about unknown sources that contribute to air pollution. Ambient concentrations of various pollutants are being monitored more systematically than in the past (especially in urban Centres). Yet very few studies have looked at personal exposures to these pollutants. There have also been few epidemiological studies to evaluate the health effects of air pollution in Indian cities. Few studies have attempted to synthesize knowledge regarding human health risks from air pollution in an integrated manner; sources of air pollution and exposure and effects, data have rarely been measured simultaneously in a single consistent experimental design.

An attempt has been made here to review the literature pertaining to salient issues in the calculation of health risks from particulate air pollution in Indian cities. The focus is on particulate air pollution because it has become increasingly clear that thoracic particulate matter (PM) is the major cause of human mortality and morbidity from air pollution. Studies in the United States (US) have indicated that there are 20,000–100,000 deaths due to particulate pollution per year *(US Environmental Protection Agency [EPA] 1996)*. Particulate pollution in Indian cities is far worse. So it is likely that per capita mortality from urban air pollution in India is at least as high as that in the US. In addition to particulate air pollution, other primary pollutants are also a cause for concern in India. The primary pollutants are (CO, nitrogen oxides, and hydrocarbons).

The main categories of urban air pollution sources in India are vehicular emissions, industrial emissions, and fuel use for domestic purposes such as cooking, and a potentially large miscellaneous category, which includes burning of household wastes, emissions from small businesses and cremation grounds. Natural sources of PM are also significant, depending on location and season. While particulates from natural sources are not conventional pollutants, their contributions are typically taken into account in inventories of total suspended particulates (TSP), since natural sources can be both a major contributor to pollution and a source of uncertainty. However, natural dust particles are coarse and do not contribute significantly to PM fractions that actually get deposited in human lungs. In Delhi, for example, dust-laden winds from the western desert during the dry season increase the TSP levels, although they have a much smaller impact on particles <10 μm in diametre.

An attempt is made here, though of-course briefly to analyze the inventions of sources of air pollution in Mumbai and Delhi. This is done only primarily to show the nature and magnitude of air pollution.

Rapid Urbanisation in India has led to an increase in transportation demand that public transport systems have been unable to meet adequately. Consequently, the use of personal vehicles has increased dramatically, between 1986 and 1991, the total number of vehicles in India increased roughly threefold, from about 9 million to 25 million, and it was estimated that the number of vehicles would reach well above 40 million by the year 2000 *(Government of India [GOI], 1993)*. Roughly half of these vehicles are in three major metropolitan cities: Delhi (~30 per cent), Mumbai (12 per cent), and Calcutta (8 per cent). Nationwide, about 70 per cent of the vehicles are gasoline-fueled personal vehicles, two- or three-wheeled vehicles that have two-stroke engines. Other gasoline-fueled vehicles, mostly cars and motorcycles with four-stroke engines, make up 14 per cent of the fleet, and diesel-fueled trucks and buses make up 8 per cent of the total.

The number of two and three-wheeled vehicles, which also represents the largest fraction of all vehicles, has been growing at the rate of 20 per cent annually and, between 1987 and 1993, increased threefold, from 7 million to 20 million. The number of two-wheelers is expected to keep rising, with a projected 36 million by 2000. Passenger cars and diesel-fueled vehicles though fewer in numbers, will double in the same time period. In the mid-1980s, the introduction of cars by Maruti, a public-sector company jointly launched by the Indian government and Suzuki of Japan, gave impetus to car purchasing by members of India's upper classes. The government's liberalisation programme, launched in the early 1990s, has encouraged car production by multinationals in India; there has been an even more dramatic rise in the number of passenger cars in the country. Recent figures showed that, between the late 1980s and 1997, the annual sales of automobiles increased >10-fold, from 40,000 to 400,000. (Chakravarti, 1998)

In keeping with the increase in numbers of vehicles, the vehicular use of gasoline and diesel fuel more than doubled over the time period of 19811994, increasing from 1.5 and 7.2 million tons, respectively, in 1981, to 3.5 and 14.8 million tons in 1994 (Agrawal *et al.* 1997). Although >80 per cent of the vehicular fleet consists of vehicles that use gasoline, the total amount of diesel fuel consumed in India exceeds the usage of gasoline by close to a factor of five. Diesel fuel is the primary fuel for buses, trucks, and other commercial vehicles, which consume larger quantities of fuel per road mile and also constitute a larger share of road miles traveled. In addition, a significant amount of diesel fuel is consumed in the generation of power by captive power plants (which supply roughly 10 per cent of the energy consumed in India). The distinction between gasoline and diesel fuel is important because, the contributions of both fuel types to multiple pollutants and air pollution health risks are significant, but the technical and policy solutions for reducing these emissions may be quite different.

The principal pollutants emitted by vehicles are carbon monoxide (CO), NOx, particulate matter (PM_{10}), volatile organic compounds, and semi-volatile poly-aromatic hydrocarbons (PAHs). Sulphur oxides are emitted in various quantities depending on the sulphur content of the fuel. Exhaust gases from gasoline-fueled vehicles also contain Lead (Pb) additives, which continue to be used although there has been a recent move toward unleaded gasoline in the major cities.

The conditions for significant Ozone pollutionthe presence of volatile organic compounds, NOx sources, abundant sunlight, and meteorological conditions such as winter inversion layersexist in many Indian cities, particularly in Delhi and Calcutta; yet the magnitude of the Ozone problem is almost entirely unknown. To our knowledge there have been no measurements of Ozone in any of the major Indian cities.

Translating numbers of vehicles to gross emissions of pollutants requires the development of representative values, called emission factors that for each vehicle category, relate the quantity of a pollutant released into the atmosphere to the level of activity associated with each vehicle type.

Emission factors are typically developed for each vehicle type, and an assessment of the variability must be performed to derive a range of values for emissions under different operating conditions. Typically, emission factors are reported for a set of ideal conditions (e.g. for a particular speed, operating temperature, and vehicular age) and with correction factors that can be used to extrapolate to other operating conditions (*US EPA AP-42 Manual*, 1985).

There are several reasons to expect larger emission factors for vehicles in India than their equivalents in industrialised countries. A majority of vehicles in India are not equipped with pollution control equipment, and only recently has the government mandated installation of catalytic converters on cars sold in the major metropolitan areas, including Mumbai and Delhi. In addition, maintenance of vehicles is poor, and there is very little monitoring and enforcement of emission standards.

Average traffic speeds, particularly in Delhi, have dropped dramatically over the past decade as vehicle density (the number of registered vehicles per square kilometer) has risen rapidly (*GOI, 1993*). The average speed of 20 km/h (TERI 1993) in Delhi is far slower than the US average of >50 km/h. Slower speeds (<30 km/h) with increased phases of acceleration and deceleration result in significantly larger emission factors than do higher cruising speeds.

Another key issue in the derivation of emission factors is the quality of fuel used. In the Indian context, the quality of fuel, especially adulteration of gasoline by kerosene, is particularly important, if understudied issue. This problem is almost universal among motorised three-wheeled vehicles (auto-rickshaws), which for the most part are not owned by their operators. Kerosene is heavily subsidised because it is seen as an important fuel for household cooking for lower-income groups. Since the price of gasoline per litre exceeds that of kerosene by a factor of five, auto-rickshaw operators typically adulterate their gasoline fuel with as much as 30 per cent kerosene. In addition, operators mix excessive amountsas much as 10 per cent (as opposed to the typical operating value of 1.5 per cent2 per cent)of lubricating oil to compensate for poor fuel quality resulting from addition of kerosene. While this can shorten engine life, the vehicles are typically not owned by the operator but rented from the owner, so there is little incentive on the part of the operators not to adulterate the fuel. Lubricating oil, which is sold in unpackaged form mainly for use in motorised two and three-wheeled vehicles, is also adulterated. Furthermore, gasoline is not the only petroleum product that is adulterated. Diesel fuel is also adulterated with kerosene, since the price of the former is almost twice that of the latter. Kerosene and lubricating oil increase emission factors, although there are few measurements of the extent to which they do so.

In the United States, the EPA has developed the infrastructure to create a regularly updated inventory of emission factor data for a wide range of vehicular and other pollutant sources (*US EPA*, 1985). However, as noted earlier, the vehicular fleet status and operating conditions in India are quite different from those in the US, and US data for the most part are not very helpful in evaluating emission factors under Indian conditions. In India, emission factor data are not as extensive and are less readily available, although some data are available from studies conducted by the Indian Institute of Petroleum and the Automotive Research Association of India. In provide a compilation of emission factors from various sources and compare them with emission factors evaluated by the US EPA.

After gaining independence in 1947, India embarked on a path of rapid industrialisation in all the major manufacturing sectorsiron and steel, heavy manufacturing, industrial and petrochemicals, and agricultural and paper products. Today, despite its label as a "less-industrialised country," India is heavily industrialised, with a thriving manufacturing sector that until recently was largely indigenous. The CPCB has catalogued over 1500 large-scale industrial units in 17 industrial categories (CPCB, 1995), accounting for about 60 per cent of India's industrial output. Small-scale industries are an important part of the Indian economy and account for the remaining 40 per cent of the industrial output. At present, India has over three million small factories (Confederation of Indian Industry, 1996).

Mumbai and Delhi are both major industrial centres with many large and small-scale industries. In addition to being India's financial and commercial capital, Mumbai is also

India's most industrialised city. The industrial belt in and around Mumbai is responsible for more than 10 per cent of India's industrial productivity, with a substantially greater fraction of the country's chemical, petrochemical, and drug manufacturing. Not surprisingly, residents of Mumbai, particularly those in the eastern suburbs where the larger industries are concentrated, face a disproportionate burden of industrial emissions. Small-scale manufacturing is also spread over the entire greater Mumbai region. Although exact numbers are hard to establish, one estimate suggests that there are 40,000 small-scale plants and big industries in the Mumbai area, of which 32 are classified as hazardous (Shah & Nagpal, 1997). Industries contributing to air pollution include textile mills, chemical and pharmaceutical engineering units, and foundries. While regulations have limited the growth of large industrial plants in the capital territory of Delhi, this has not affected the growth of number of small-scale units. Small-scale manufacturing units in Delhi include everything from metalworking to food processing. One estimate places the number of small-scale units at 93,000 (CPCB, 1993).

Industries emit a wide variety of process-specific pollutantsgaseous organic and inorganic compounds, complex vapours that undergo phase transformation after emission into the atmosphere, and PM with process-specific composition (e.g. heavy metals and PAHs). The presence of a large number of small-scale industrial plants makes pollution control more difficult because, small-scale operations are more financially strapped and less technologically capable than large-scale ones, and their numbers make the already lax monitoring and enforcement of pollution control laws even more difficult.

Criterion pollutants (SOx, NOx, CO, HC, and PM) that are released as a part of industrial combustion may be quantified to the first order on the basis of overall estimates of fuel used and average emission factors for various industrial activities. Determination of the levels of specific toxic substances released into the environment, on the other hand, requires plant-specific data for each toxic compound. Construction of inventories for specific chemicals is a resource-intensive and difficult activity owing to its process-specific nature. Detailed inventories for each industry and each plant can be calculated only through regular monitoring of emissions. Curiously, while a catastrophic industrial disaster in Indiathe Bhopal tragedywas the catalyst for enactment of the Emergency Planning and Community-Right-to-Know Act (EPCRA) in the US, leading to the creation of a Toxics Release Inventory (TRI), such databases are not available for India. The result is that data for estimating industrial emissions are sparse.

While it is a safe assumption that Mumbai and Delhi have substantial emissions of toxic substances and heavy metals, many small towns also may have local manufacturing units with potentially high-level toxic emissions. For example, Moradabad, a small town in the state of Uttar Pradesh, is a Centre for brass production (smelting, electroplating, cutting, scraping, and machining), and ambient measurements there have revealed very high levels of heavy metals such as Pb, Cd, Cu, and Zn (Tripathi *et al.*, 1989). It is likely that many other places face similar localised issues regarding the release of toxic substances.

One consequence of the lack of detailed inventories and the heterogeneity of emissions is that simple scaling of information from one situation cannot be used to determine industrial emissions in another situation. In the rest of our discussion of industrial emissions we will construct an inventory of emissions from two categoriespower plants and other industriesfor Mumbai and Delhi.

Coal-fired power plants generate two-thirds of India's electric power (GOI 1996). Its coal-fired power capacity is expected to grow from 55 GW in 1996 to 80 GW by 2002. Indian steam coal is high in ash content (30 per cent50 per cent) but low in sulfur (<0.5 per cent). More than 99 per cent of the coal used in the generation of electric power in India is domestic steam coal. Additionally, the ash is very high in silica and aluminum (>90 per cent). This results in very high resistivity for the fly ash (10^{13} to 10^{15} -cm), which makes it difficult for conventional electrostatic precipitators (ESPs) to collect fly ash efficiently (Lookman & Rubin, 1998). Conventional ESPs are the only devices used in Indian power plants for control of PM; thus, more efficient pre- and post-combustion methods such as coal washing and the use of flue gas conditioning are not being applied. Existing efficiencies of ESPs of 85 per cent95 per cent result in emissions of >45 million tons of fly ash from Indian power plants each year (Confederation of Indian Industry 1996). The main method of disposal of fly ash from power stations is mixing it with water; the resultant slurry is pumped through pipes to ash disposal ponds. Coal combustion in thermal power plants also emits a variety of toxic heavy metals, such as Pb, Zn, Ni, Co, Cd, Cr, and Cu.

Delhi has three power plants, all coal fired, located within its city limits: the 235-MW Indraprastha Power Station (IPP station); the 135-MW Rajghat Power House, and the 720-MW Badarpur Thermal Power Station (BTPS). The total quantity of fly ash from the three power plants is about 6000 tons per day (Indraprastha 12001500, Rajghat 600800, and Badarpur 35004000 tons per day [GOI 1997]). In these power plants, ash is collected by ESPs which have collection efficiencies that are higher than average for India99.3 per cent (IPP station), 99.7 per cent (Rajghat Power House), and 98 per cent (BTPS) (Mehra *et al.*, 1998). Nonetheless, there are episodes of major particulate pollution around the power stations from fly ash dispersal. The larger IPP plant also has shorter stacks (60 m) than the Rajghat Power House plant (160 m) and thus is more likely to cause human PM exposures. We calculated PM_{10} emissions from power plants in Delhi by using the above estimates for fly ash production and a range for ESP collection efficiency of 97.5 per cent99.5 per cent. The resulting estimate for PM_{10} emissions is between 45,000 and 125,000 tons/year.

In contrast, Mumbai has one major thermal power plant, the Tata thermal plant, located in the industrial eastern section of the city. In addition, a 360-MW nuclear power plant is also located near Mumbai, in Tarapur. The Tata thermal station has a total generation capacity of 1 GW (2 units of 500 MW) and can use multiple fuel typescoal, natural gas, and oilwith typical usage of these fuels in the ratio of 1:2:3. Ash and PM are collected by ESPs, and at 278 m the plant's stacks are tall.

The URBAIR study (Shah & Nagpal, 1997) estimated that the total PM_{10} emitted from power plants in Mumbai is roughly 1500 tons/year. This is considerably less than the estimate for Delhi, and partly because the Delhi power plants are completely coal based whereas the TATA thermal plant uses coal for only one-fifth of its fuel needs. The rest of the fuel requirement is met by using distillate oil and gas. Furthermore, the URBAIR study uses US emission factors, which may underestimate emissions in India by an order of magnitude. The particulate emission limit for Indian power plants is set at 150 mg/Nm^3, although the general level of compliance is acknowledged to be poor. By contrast, in the United States, the New Source Performance Standard is 30 mg/Nm^3 while the current best-practice level is roughly 5 mg/Nm^3 (Lookman & Rubin, 1998). We assume that the per-megawatt PM_{10} emissions from coal-based power in Mumbai are the same as in Delhi, and PM_{10} emissions from Mumbai are estimated to be in the range of 700020,000 tons per year.

Particulate emissions resulting from industrial combustion of fossil fuels have been characterised for Mumbai and Delhi in some studies shows levels of PM_{10} emissions by power plants and other industries in these two cities, estimated by three different studies besides this one. For Delhi, while the three other studies have different estimates of total emissions, they show roughly equal contributions by power plants and other industries to PM_{10} emissions. A GOI white paper (GOI, 1997) on air pollution in Delhi also estimated that PM_{10} emissions from other industries were roughly equal to power plant emissions. There is insufficient information on the assumptions that went into the inventory calculations of the two other studies (CPCB, 1994; Saxena & Dayal, 1997).

A number of diseases have been associated with inhalation exposure to airborne PM: respiratory disorders whose effects range from minor symptoms such as coughs and dyspnea to severe ones such as acute respiratory infections (ARI), asthma, and pneumonia, chronic obstructive lung diseases such as bronchitis, cardiovascular disease, tuberculosis, lung cancer, and blindness. In addition, peri-natal effects such as still births and low birth weights are also associated with air pollution. However, the health end point that is most clearly defined is death, and many epidemiological studies in developed countries focus on obtaining relationships between mortality rates and ambient levels of pollution.

High levels of chronic morbidity exact their own toll and pose severe strains on the health care infrastructure. For instance, one study estimated that the incidence of respiratory diseases in Delhi is 12-fold higher than that for the rest of the country. A preliminary study of a middle-class population in East Delhi also found that 23 per cent of the population suffered from severe respiratory disorders and 54 per cent of the population suffered from some form of respiratory disease (Pandey, 1998). The study also found that the sale of drugs that help combat respiratory disease, like Citrizine (an antihistamine), Salbutamol (a bronchial dilator), Bromzine (mucolactice; liquifies sputum), Amoxicillin, and Erythromycin (antibiotics for respiratory tract infections), is increasing at the rate of 20 per cent per year, which is much faster than the current rate of population growth.

As for other parts of the causal paradigm, very few epidemiological studies have been conducted on the health risks of exposure to PM in Indian cities. Much of the science of exposure and effects assessment has been developed in industrialised countries, particularly the US. This understanding is routinely relied upon for making extrapolations to other contexts, such as India, where the science is less well studied. For example, several assessments of mortality from air pollution in India use simple reduced-form expressions, derived from US studies, linking mortality to PM concentration. There are good reasons to believe that the science developed in one context may be applicable in others. Certainly the prevailing scientific view is that epidemiological studies performed in regions with similar levels and types of exposure, demographics, and statuses of public health result in findings of similar effects and human mortality in these regions. However, the differences between urban India and industrialised settings like the US are large enough that extrapolations of US findings to India are likely to produce misleading analyses. This could result in errors in aggregate calculations of human mortality, in the magnitude of health risks faced by specific vulnerable groups, and ultimately in analysing the ways in which exposure reduction can be achieved.

While socioeconomic factors are also important confounders, very few studies have looked at them systematically. Again, the study by Kamat (1984) provides some evidence of the importance of these factors. Of the four communities studied, the rural area had the lowest level of outdoor air pollution, but it showed an intermediate degree of morbidity. The villages studied typically had no sanitation, no protected water supply, poor housing, poor nutrition, widespread intestinal parasitism, and poor quality of medical care. These factors, over a long period of time, may have accounted for the poorer health status and lung function of the residents. (Mishra *et al.*, (1997) showed that persons living in households with a separate kitchen had lower risks of tuberculosis than persons living in houses without a separate kitchen. Educational levels were also found to be strongly linked to tuberculosis prevalence. These findings are unlike observations from studies conducted in the West (Mostardi & Leonard, 1974; Ferris *et al.*, 1979); those studies show no effect of socioeconomic status on lung function or other measures of health status.

A number of authors, however, argue that exposure to PM is an important determinant of mortality, even when socioeconomic status is taken into account. Globally, ARI is a major cause of infant mortality, killing 4.3 million children per year (WHO, 1992). ARI is the single largest disease category in India, accounting for one-eighth of the national disease burden (Smith, 1999). In a Brazilian study, Penna & Duchiade (1991) observed statistically significant associations between average annual levels of PM and infant mortality from pneumonia after controlling for socioeconomic factors such as family income level. Researchers in Kerala have also found an association between pneumonia, a number of socioeconomic variables, and air pollution (Shah *et al.*, 1994). Smith (1993) summarised studies conducted in five different lesser-developed countries which indicated that the relative risk for severe ARI from smoke exposures might be in the range of two to six. Clearly, socioeconomic status and exposure to air pollution are heavily linked in India. In this work, we analyze this linkage by studying the effects of income on exposure and, consequently, on health. (Reference: Annual Review of Energy and the Environment Vol. 25: 629-684 (Volume publication date November 2000) (Milind Kandlikar, Department of Engineering and Public Policy, Carnegie Mellon University, Pittsburgh, Pennsylvania

15213, Gurumurthy Ramachandran- Division of Environmental and Occupational Health, School of Public Health, University of Minnesota, Minneapolis, Minnesota 55455)

Half of the world's households use biomass fuels, including wood, animal dung, or crop residues, that produce wide-array toxic particles, carbon monoxide, and other indoor pollutants. The World Health Organisation (WHO) has determined that as many as 1 billion people, mostly women and children, are regularly exposed to levels of indoor air pollution that are up to 100 times those considered acceptable. Young children, who spend more time indoors, are more exposed to the noxious byproducts of cooking and heating. In India, where 80 *per cent* of households use biomass fuel, estimates show that nearly 500,000 women and children under age 5 die every year from indoor pollution, largely from acute respiratory infections (ARIs). The figure for other less developed countries is similar.

Exposure to indoor pollutants can cause or aggravate ARIs, including upper respiratory infections such as colds and sore throats, and lower respiratory infections such as pneumonia. Acute lower respiratory infections are one of the primary causes of child mortality in developing countries, and led to 2.2 million deaths in children under age 5 in 2001. ARIs can also increase mortality from measles, malaria, and other diseases. Other factors that can worsen ARIs include low birth weight, poor nutrition, inadequate housing and poor hygiene conditions, overcrowding, and reduced access to health care.

Asthma Studies in less developed countries have linked indoor air pollution to lung cancer, stillbirths, low birth weight, heart ailments, and chronic respiratory diseases, including asthma.

Data suggest that over 60 *per cent* of the diseases associated with respiratory infections are linked to exposure to air pollution. Outdoor pollutants such as sulfur dioxide, ozone, nitrogen oxide, carbon monoxide, and volatile organic compounds come mainly from motor vehicle exhaust, power plant emissions, open burning of solid waste, and construction and related activities.

Contaminated water and inadequate sanitation cause a range of diseases, many of which are life-threatening. The most deadly are diarrheal diseases, 80 *per cent* to 90 *per cent* of which result from environmental factors. In 2001, diarrheal infections caused nearly 2 million deaths in children under age 5, primarily due to dehydration; many more children suffer from non-fatal diarrhea that leaves them underweight, physically stunted, vulnerable to disease and drained of energy. Poor sanitation conditions and inadequate personal, household and community hygiene are responsible for most of diarrheal infections.

Despite significant investments in improving water supplies and sanitation over the last 20 years, about 18 *per cent* of the World's population still lacks access to safe drinking water, and nearly 40 *per cent* have no access to sanitation.

In developing countries, the poorest strata are often excluded from the benefits of emerging prosperity and may also face a disproportionate share of health risks related to economic growth. Urban slums may be located near major roads, factories, or dumpsites, for instance, exposing residents to higher levels of air pollution or to the risks of industrial accidents. The chief victims of the accident at Bhopal, India, for example, were not just workers but slum dwellers who had settled near the factory.

Looking ahead at development, environment, and health, then, it seems vital to consider distribution of wealth as well as rising income. Economic growth in and of itself is not sufficient to improve health for all, especially if rising income disparities mean that millions of people will not participate in these advances. As this income gap increases, the health gap is also likely to grow, leading to what some have dubbed "epidemiologic polarisation." Unlike the more optimistic scenario of a smooth transition to better health, with a dramatic decline in infectious disease, this polarisation scenario foresees a future in which mortality from infectious disease and malnutrition remains high but is increasingly concentrated among the poor. As WHO reported in 1997, many countries are already experiencing this polarisation. (The World Resources Institute - Poverty, Health, and the Environment. World Resources – 1998-99)

Nature of Environmental Pollution in Bangalore City

Having discussed the impact of Urbanisation on environment by drawing on the evidence in two mega cities Mumbai and Delhi, let us turn to Bangalore city–growth of Bangalore city and the concomitant growth of slum and slum population have been discussed in the previous chapter.

Bangalore city has become increasingly the most polluted city in India. Air pollution is increasingly at an alarming rate and it is solely due to constant smoke emanating from vehicles plying on the road. Quality of air has deteriorated beyond permissible limits.

Air Pollution

According to the report published by (WHO) World Health Organisation, United Nations Environment Programme, air pollution is the most serious threat to the life of people living in urban areas. Health disorders caused by air pollutants depend upon and determined by the intensity, duration of exposure. The pollutants directly affect the respiratory digestive nerves and cardiovascular systems. Increased incidents of death, disease and disability have been associated with elevated levels of SO_2, SPM, RPM and CO displaces Oxygen in the blood. It causes severe headache, dizziness, nausea, mental retardation and neurological disorders, NO and O_3 affect seriously the respiratory system, irritate eyes, nose and throat. Lead content in the air causes bone marrow; obstruct liver, heart and kidney functions. So much so, there is increasing evidence which suggest a link between increasing air pollution and increase in the incidents heart attack. All types of vehicles are seen on Bangalore city roads and they have been classified as follows: Two-wheelers like scooter, mopeds and motor-cycles, followed by three-wheelers that is auto-rickshaw, four-wheelers like cars, buses and lorries and a host of other trucks. Of these vehicles, two-wheelers are a menace, because of their high density and defective engine design. Among many busy roads in Bangalore city, the road from Ananda Rao circle to Mahathama Gandhi circle, from there to Trinity circle and from Anand Rao circle via K.R. circle leading to Corporation circle are the busiest roads. The movement of two-wheelers is very high. One of the reasons for high density of vehicles is lack of dependable efficient and sufficient public transport system. More than 60 per cent of the population depend upon their own vehicles that too two-wheelers.

Trinity circle: Trinity circle has the highest vehicular density and as a result it has high RPM level in the ambient air (393mg/m3). At the site, petrol driven vehicles, 2-3 wheelers and light duty four wheelers are more pronounced compared to other sampling sites.

K.R. circle: K.R. circle has the second highest vehicular density and the RPM concentration was 374mg/m3. The lead concentration is 0.90mg/m3 at site petrol and diesel driven vehicles are much more in number.

Anand Rao circle: Anand Rao circle takes up third place in lead concentration and RPM concentration is 307mg/m3. This is due to many factors. The temperature recorded at Anand Rao circle is much more than what prevails at trinity circle (340C). Due to high wind speed and temperature the pollutant tend to get dispersed.

K.R.Market: K.R.Market comes fourth in lead concentration and RPM was 273mg/m3. At market place the roads are too narrow and highly congested.

Jaya Nagara circle: Whereas at Jaya Nagar the roads are wider. Tall buildings live on both side of the roads there is enough scope for dispersion of pollutants. Vegetation present in Jaya Nagara is acting as a trap for the pollutants, whereas at the market absence of vegetation might be the reason for the more RPM concentration (256mg/m3).

V.V.Puram circle: At V.V.Puram circle the roads are wider and tall trees live on both sides of the roads. The volume of traffic generally high yet flows smoothly the RPM concentration was 153mg/m3. In the city limits, the permissible noise limit from horns is 91 decibels (dB). "There are four zones, residential, commercial, and industrial and the sensitive zone. The sensitive zone includes areas where there are hospitals and schools," according to a senior official of the Karnataka State Pollution Control Board (KSPCB).

Noise Pollution

Since air horns exceed the permissible decibel limit, they are banned by government policy. "Particularly in the last five years, there has been increase in awareness about noise levels and, therefore, none of the BMTC buses use air horns. Once in three months, the BMTC buses are checked in the depots and the horn is one of the things that is checked," says the KSPCB official.

But private travel operators use air horns. At the time of getting the vehicle checked for the fitness certificate every year, these operators change the bus horns and after the check-up, they install air horns again, says the official. It is noticed that the buses traveling towards Anekal, Kunigal, Tumkur, Magadi and other places use blaring air horns. Sharma Travels admits that their fleet of 64 buses use air horns but outside city limits on the highway. "However, within city limits, we use only electric horns," says Mr H R Srinivasan, Works Manager at Sharma Transport. Mr Badrinath of Sri Satya Sai Tourists says that only their interstate buses are fitted with air horns. National Travels also says that air horns are used only outside city limits and are used sparingly. Transport Commissioner I M Vittal Murthy clarifies that air horns are not allowed within and outside city limits.

The special drive has a two-fold objective - to create awareness and check noise pollution. There are 25 police squads stationed in different areas of Bangalore to check pollution of any kind, including noise pollution, says Mr Murthy. However, a handicap faced by the department is the absence of sound metres to gauge the noise levels. It is long pending and the department officials and inspectors continue to check noise levels with their ears!

The department also finds it difficult to book cases against noisy vehicles due to the lack of parameters to judge them. "Vehicles need to possess the 'Under Control Certificate' for air pollution, but there's isn't an equivalent for noise pollution," he says. But, till the department concerned decides to control and manage noise on the roads, spread of awareness seems to be the answer to control noise. "During the training sessions, we are taught about safety and also about saving fuel. We are also told that we should not use the horn near hospitals and schools," says Anil Kumar, BMTC driver (Route No. 171).

The first step towards controlling noise pollution through blaring horns is to wait for the vehicle in front of you to move before you blow the horn. Remember that there is someone behind honking at you as well. (Suma Tekur, Deccan Herald 26th January, 2004, The Printers (Mysore) Private Ltd)

The Transport Department recently flagged off a 'courtesy month' in the city to create some awareness among citizens about vehicles, pollution, etc. Given the multiplicity of vehicles on the roads and the absence of road and traffic sense, how far will this drive succeed?

Major contributors to noise pollution include buses, lorries, vehicles with shrill horns and autorickshaws, some of which ply without (or with altered) sound mufflers in the silencers, apparently for better speed and mileage! While Bangaloreans with their 'swalpa adjust maadi' attitude have simply learnt to put up with such noise, visitors feel the autos are noisy and irritating.

Adulterated fuel used by the auto drivers does not burn the fuel completely and leaves a residue of unburned hydrocarbon which chokes the silencers and reduces the performance of the vehicle. Ramesh H, a mechanic at Shivajinagar says, since auto drivers usually run hired vehicles, they mix kerosene to petrol which is economical. To curb such practices, the government allowed use of chemicals with kerosene meant for auto consumption (popularly known as blue kerosene). However, this fuel is known to cause damage to the engine, but continues to be used as most drivers can't afford petrol, Ramesh said. According to S B Rao, an engineer at the Bajaj Research and Development Centre, Pune, autos which roll out of the manufacturing units produce noise in accordance with levels permitted under the Central Motor Vehicles Act, while those fitted with modified silencers produce about three times more noise.

The modified silencers, which are locally made and go by the reference 'dolly silencers', are easily available in City Market area. Ram Murthy a shop owner here says, these modifiers have turned out to be very economical. However, they have contributed greatly to the noise levels in the City. Bangalore is believed to be experiencing six times more noise than permitted levels and authorities are contemplating mandatory noise emission tests. Meanwhile, the Transport Department is gearing up to tackle increasing noise pollution. Transport Commissioner I M Vittal Murthy admitted that the police are not equipped with devices to detect the extra noise produced by vehicles. "The RTO checks the vehicles for modified silencers during their permit renewals. The drivers use the normal silencers at that time and change it later. The noise on the roads hampers the process to check any extra noise. The only option is to educate the drivers and I think such programmes will change the mindset of the offenders." He noted that the reason why the present campaign stresses on public participation is because campaigns only by the government don't have the targeted impact.

A large number of NGOs, student unions, NSS, NCC cadets, artists and celebrities will lend their support. An oath to protect the environment will be administered to school and college students, apart from several competitions. "With our slogan 'I love my Bangalore and I will keep it clean', we hope to create a strong enough impact on violators to mend their ways," he said. The last day of the 'courtesy month' will witness a human chain by students and volunteers on the Outer Ring Road. Fifty artists from 'Parisarakkagi Kalavidaru' have started painting environment-related themes and slogans on BMTC and KSRTC buses. Twenty-five police squads at strategic points will impose mild penalties on traffic violators in the first week and heavier fines from second week onwards. (Pravin D. Shiriyannavar)

Noise is not a very visible form of pollution. Increasingly, we are being assaulted by higher and higher decibel levels, leading to a concomitant rise in stress levels. Sonira Gulhati checks out an urban menace that is not being taken seriously.

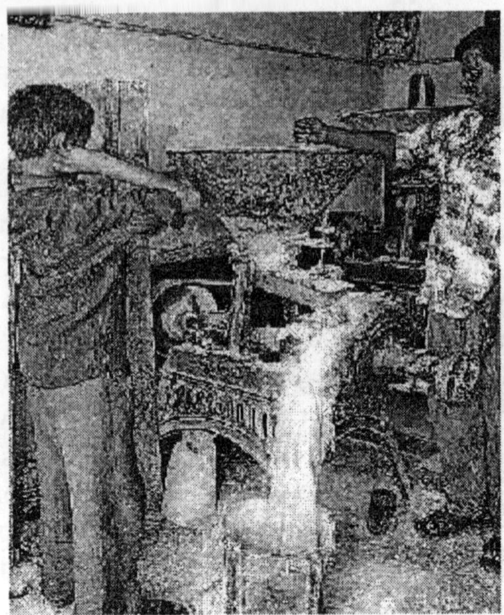

Figure – 1

The pulveriser makes too loud a racket for this young customer

When did you last experience something called peaceful silence? When you could hear only the insects chirruping or the gentle rustle of leaves? Well, leaves (what's left of them) and insects (what's left of them) are still around, but what has overwhelmed their gentle presence is man-made - noise. Try and watch a movie on TV with sparkling dialogues, and nine times out of ten, you will miss the crucial bits, thanks to the passing roar of a truck in second gear or the irritating whine of an auto-rickshaw running on adulterated fuel. As for that blender making all that racket in the kitchen, it is in strong competition with that ghetto blaster your kid has put on, though his room is closed.

Silence is golden. It has also become a thing of the past for the urban dweller. As cities grow in size and population, it is becoming increasingly difficult for quiet to prevail.

Bangalore, being a large growing city, has over 20 lakh vehicles. Traffic is a major factor in creating unwanted noise. It's not just the noise of the internal combustion engine that is part of the traffic noise, those who control them also add their bit by leaning on the horns every 10 seconds, something unheard of in other countries.

And how many of you have cursed auto-rickshaws whose silencers have been removed, multiplying the decibel level, forcing you to contemplate homicide? Not only are these vehicles badly designed in every way, their drivers often remove the noise mufflers in the belief that it improves pick-up.

Apart from this kind of noise pollution, there are others like that from loud speakers, generators, construction site equipment, bore-well rigs, and so on. All these and more have a deleterious effect on the City dweller's health.

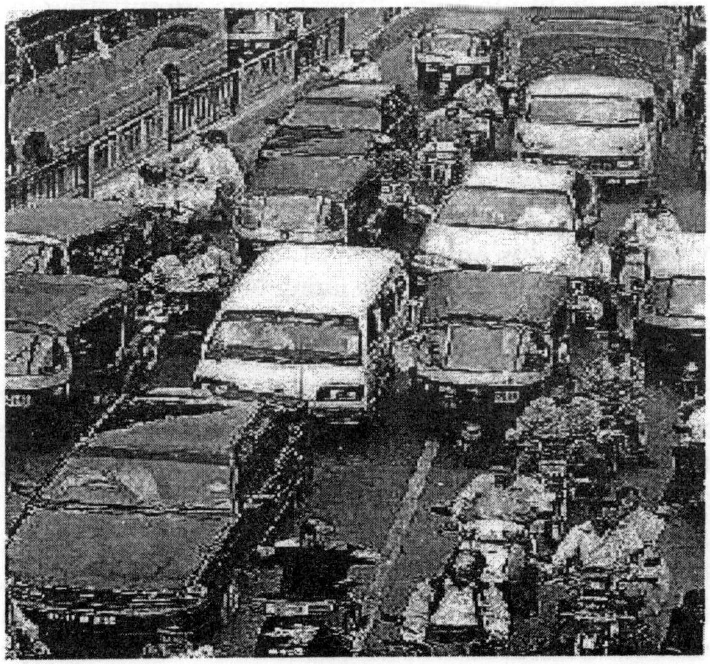

Figure- 2

Traffic noise adds to stress levels, which is detrimental to everyone's health.

Noise pollution adds to stress levels and in the long run, has been proved to damage our hearing faculties. The louder the noise one is exposed to over a continued period of time, the faster it leads to hearing loss.

Says Dr. G. Mohan, ENT surgeon, Mallya Hospital: "The levels of noise in the City have definitely gone up. The vehicular noise doesn't so much cause damage to hearing but increases stress levels and causes irritability. But prolonged exposure to certain kinds of industrial noise can cause damage to the inner ear and eventually to the nerve cells located there." Unlike other forms of pollution that assault the eyes and the nose, noise pollution is invisible. With the fast-paced city life, urban dwellers have no time to pause and think about the knocking their other senses are taking, thanks to noise. Bangaloreans are suffering the effects of noise through increasing volume of traffic. Moreover, the quality of traffic is steadily deteriorating. In a day and age when everything is instant, patience has become obsolete among drivers. Says Nitya Mohan, a resident of Ulsoor: "There is no longer decorum on the roads. People are just in too much of a hurry and have lost any sensitivity towards fellow citizens." The problem of unwanted noise affects people living in the central parts of the City as well as those living in what were once quiet areas. Says Krishna Srinivasan, a resident of Dollar Colony, a secluded area: "It used to be quite different when we moved here in the '80s. Now even though we are more than a kilometre away from the main Bellary Road, we can hear the noise of the trucks and other vehicles."

There are laws against noise pollution, and Bangalore has a Pollution Control Board that is very much functional. B. Ramaiah, Senior Environment officer of the Karnataka State Pollution Control Board blames industries for the increasing level of noise in the City. "The increasing number of offices and industries has added to the noise levels in the City. Offices use captive generators that create a lot of noise," he adds.

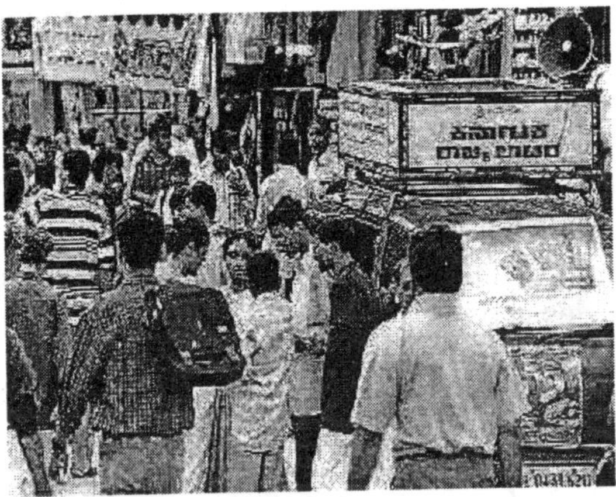

Figure – 3

Adding to the decibel level are the loudspeakers, either advertising products or haranguing the public.

The World Health Organisation's guidelines recommend a night-time average level suitable for undisturbed sleep from 35 to 30 decibels (dB), including a peak night-time maximum of 45 dB. In most large cities the average night-time noise levels exceed 45 to 50 dB. The Indian Environment Protection Act prescribes a certain maximum level of sound that is allowed under the law. "In industrial areas, the maximum allowed limit is 75dB in the day and about 70dB at night. Similarly, in residential areas the (permitted) limit is about 65dB in the day and 60dB at night, and in areas which qualify as silent zones, like areas surrounding hospitals, the prescribed upper limit is about 55dB in the day and 45dB at night," says Mr. Ramaiah.

In cases of bore well drilling at night-time, use of loud speakers or any noise created intentionally by a third party, every citizen is protected under the Environmental Protection Act and has a right to seek help. "Every citizen is protected against noise and has the right to seek help against anybody who is creating noise that is disturbing and illegal. The local police station must immediately be informed and action will be taken," he adds.

According to research, noise intensities above 55 dB are enough to cause annoyance and aggressive behaviour. Also, noise above 75 dB can lead to increased stress levels, increased heart rates and potential hearing loss.

A recent study by two engineering students in the City on noise levels at two major traffic junctions turned up alarming statistics. Most buses, auto-rickshaws, and motorcycles grossly exceeded the noise level, with one of the buses touching as much as 100 dB. On M.G. Road, the levels were as much at 82.5 dB. With society becoming noisier than ever, it is up to each one of us to do our bit in taking pre-emptive measures. Otherwise, we will soon turn into a society of noisy yet deaf people! The time to start is now. Is there anyone listening?

Water Pollution

Bangalore increasingly turning into 'garbage city' water pollution has among else two dimensions: contamination of fresh water bodies and ground water-depleting water resources.

Spatial Analyses in Bangalore City:

The results showed about 4.5 per cent (49.56 sq. km.) of the total area studied (1102 sq. km.) covered by water bodies. Further analysis showed a decrease of 133 water bodies (North - 42, South - 91) over a period of twenty three years, owing to pressures from public spirited endeavours, such as the public utility bus stand (e.g., Kampamudhi, Doddamudhi tanks), residential layouts, commercial establishments, stadium, recreation, etc.

Loss of water tanks in and around Bangalore City:

a) BANNERGHATTA TANK:

The **'Deepakanalla tank'** is located in the Bannerghatta

National Park in the southern part of Bangalore city. The tank is situated amidst the forest, covering an area of about five hectares. It is a major water source for the wild animals of the forest and also serves as an habitat for Indian crocodiles, varieties of fishes, birds and other microscopic form of life. The tank has no major identified point source of pollution.

The water was largely clear with non-objectionable odor through out the study period. The temperature of the water ranged from 21°-29°C (26.1± 2.6°C) and transparency ranging from 30-50 Cms and low turbidity values further support the clarity of the water body.

The pHs of the water body were found to be alkaline throughout the study period ranging from 8.1 - 9.7 which could be attributed mainly due to the dissolved substances and the geology of the area. The Electrical Conductivity was found to range from 0.20 ± 0.06 mili Siemens/cm The Dissolved Oxygen (DO) of the lake ranged from 6.0-7.0 mg/L, and the Biological Oxygen Demand (BOD) and the Chemical Oxygen Demand (COD) was shown ranging from 2 ± 0.79 mg/L and 19.4 ± 7.2 mg/L respectively.

The Suspended Solids during the entire study period ranged from 20-132mg/L with higher values noticed during the July-Sept'97 mostly be due to rain. Similar trends were noticed with the Total Solids which were found ranging from 78 - 242 mg/L and the Total Dissolved Solids were found at 93.8 ± 27.7mg/L. Among the major captions analyses, Calcium was found to range from 25.2 ± 12.25mg/L, Magnesium at 6.54 ±3.69 mg/L, Potassium values at 4.0 ± 2.7mg/L and Sodium at 34.5 ± 7.1 mg/L indicating no source of either domestic or industrial pollution. The relatively higher values of Calcium and Sodium could be due to the geo-morphology of the area. The various heavy metals that included copper, lead, iron, zinc, nickel, cadmium and chromium were found at non-detectable levels.

b) SANKEY TANK

Sankey tank is situated in the western part of the city and was constructed by Col. Sankey during the later half of the 19th Century to meet the needs and demands of Bangaloreans. Presently the tank has a well maintained park and a city corporation swimming pool to the south of the tank, and a forest department nursery towards the north of the tank. The tank provides recreation by providing boating facilities by the KSTDC (Karnataka State Tourism Development Corporation) and fishing activities, attracts birds. The tank has no major identified point source of pollution.

The water colour through out the study period was noticed to be clear with non-objectionable odour. The temperature of the water body ranged from 21° C to 30 °C during summer. The water clarity indicated by low turbidity values ranged from 6 - 14 NTU and high transparency over 25 cms.

The pH of the water samples during the entire study period was mostly neutral at all points ranging from 7.2 - 8.4. The Electrical Conductivity of water samples at Centre and outlet were 0.49 (± 0.05) and 0.55 (± 0.29) mS/cm. The higher values were noted during Apr'97 at outlet mainly from the nursery side towards outlet. The water samples showed lower Solids during the study period. The Total Solids ranged from 260 - 446 mg/L towards inlet, 264 - 398 mg/L towards Centre and 276 - 408 mg/L at the outlet. Lower Dissolved Solids of 228 (± 47.75), 234.18 (±30.97), 247.2 (±42.8) mg/L were found at inlet, Centre and outlet respectively. Similarly low values Suspended Solids at all sample points indicated that the tank has less suspended particles and pollution load.

The dissolved salts of carbonate and bicarbonates of divalent cat ions (such as Calcium and Magnesium) cause the hardness in water. Relatively higher values at about 150mg/L of total hardness were found at inlet, which may be due to runoff from the nonpoint source or the geology, (which use hardness inducing substances such as lime). The Dissolved Oxygen of the lake are at 6.6±0.9 mg/L, 6.7±0.9 mg/L and 6.6±1.0 mg/L at inlet, Centre and outlet of the tank respectively. The DO at all sample points of the lake, showed nearly same values all through the study period. Lower values of Biological Oxygen Demand ranging from 1.7 - 7.0 mg/L were noticed at all points in the lake, which clearly showed low degree of pollution. Low values of Chemical Oxygen Demand ranging from 15-105mg/L at inlet, 14-94 mg/L and 12-112 mg/L at inlet, Centre and outlet respectively clearly shows the water in this lake is relatively less polluted. Calcium values varied from 31.0 - 118.0 mg/L at various points measured in the tank. Low values of Potassium were observed from 2.0-11.0 mg/L.

c) MADIVALA TANK:

Madivala tank, the second biggest in Bangalore, only next to Bellandur tank is situated in B.T.M. layout between Bannerghatta and Hosur roads to the south of the city, covering an area of about 115 hectares. This tank has a park and a boating club provided by KSTDC for recreational purpose. It receives voluminous amounts of untreated sewage of both domestic (mainly) and industrial (mostly small scale industries) which includes dye, washings etc from surrounding areas.

The colour of the water was found green for most time during the study period mainly due to higher plankton density. During Sept-Oct'97 water was clear due to dilution on account of rain. The water temperature was between 21°C (during Dec'96-Jan'97) to 29°C (Apr-May'97).

The pH of the water samples of the tank was mostly alkaline ranging from 7.2 to 9.1. The Electrical Conductivity varied from 0.7 - 1.3 mS/cm at the various points analysed in the lake mainly due to higher dissolved solids. The Total Solids averaged at 464.3 mg/L (S.D 71.5) at inlet, 396.9 (S.D 68.9) at outlet, 321.4 (S.D 112) at Centre of the lake. Higher values of TDS were noticed at both outlet and inlet during Apr-May'97 due to decreased water level. The Dissolved Oxygen concentration throughout the study period didn't vary much from one station to another and ranged from 1.8 to 8.0 mg/L, 2.3 to 8.2 mg/L and 2.6 to 8.3 mg/L at inlet, Centre and outlet respectively. Low DO values noticed during Feb-Apr'97 were mostly due to water hyacinth. The Biological Oxygen Demand values of water samples ranged from 4.0 to 42.0mg/L towards the outlet and inlet. The higher values noticed during May-Jul'97 were mostly due to water hyacinth blooms, sewage and precipitation runoff. Organic and inorganic chemical pollution in water samples are reflected by high values of Chemical Oxygen Demand. The values in lake water samples ranged from 46.2 mg/L to 282.0 mg/L. The higher values of noticed during May-July'97 could be due to the sewage, surface runoff and by detergents from washing activities by washermen.

The Total hardness of water samples were 206 ± 34.4 mg/L at inlet, 181.7 ± 29.3 mg/L at Centre and 199.3 ± 29.4mg/L at outlet during the study period. This high value of hardness is due to domestic sewage and washing activities that takes place in the tank bed. The high Chloride contents of averaged 134.8 mg/L and is an evidence of organic pollution mainly from the domestic sources pollution and detergents. The Calcium content of the water sample indicated a decrease from 33.6 to 50.5 mg/L during Nov'96-Jan'97 and increased during Feb-Apr'97. Potassium and Magnesium are at 22.5±6.0 mg/l to 26.1±7.4 mg/L respectively.

d) HEBBAL TANK

Hebbal tank is situated in the Northern part of the city covering an area of about 75 hectares. Being one of the biggest tanks in Bangalore, it supports agricultural and fishing activities and a water source for the forest nursery adjacent the tank. The tank receives untreated domestic sewage from B.E.L layout, Vidyaranayapura, Hebbal and the surrounding areas apart from vehicular pollution of the traffic on national highway (NH-7). The tank is ecologically important as it supports a large population of migratory birds, which includes egrets, crane, coodles, kingfisher, etc. The tank, once a major drinking water source to the surrounding area is at the verge of death due to pollution.

The colour of the water body was dark grey towards the inlet (due to the sewage), greenish towards Centre and outlet (mostly from plankton). Higher values of turbidity were noticed at the Centre and inlet is due to plankton and sewage. Transparency ranges from 9.0 -22.0 cms at various points in the tank indicating low light penetration. Temperature of the water during sampling time (10-12am) ranged from 20 - 30 °C.

The pH of the tank was found mostly in alkaline region ranging from 7.5 to 8.9.The higher pH noticed could be attributed to the characteristics of the incoming sewage and plankton activity. Plankton activities increase pH by making use of the available carbon-dioxide. The Electrical Conductivity was found to be high, ranging from 1.2 to 1.5 ms/cm. higher values were noticed during the months of Apr-Jul'97 which could be due to high dissolved solids from sewage and reduced volume of water due to evaporation. The decreased values noticed during Sept-Oct'97 could be attributed to the dilution on account of runoff from the rains. The main source for Total Solids in Hebbal tank is sewage inflow, and surface run-off and were found to range from 600 - 968 mg/L at inlet, 702 - 766. mg/L at Centre and 556 - 902 mg/L at outlet. A high value at inlet was mainly due to sewage and agricultural run-off. The Dissolved Solids showed higher values at all point 514.5 ± 172.1 mg/L, 548 ± 199.7 mg/L, 485.6 ± 143.6 mg/L at inlet, Centre and outlet respectively. The steep fall in the values of dissolved solids during Aug'97 was due to increased water levels from rain and may be due to sampling done towards the periphery of the tank owing to non-availability of the boat.

All through the study period low values of Dissolved Oxygen were noticed at the inlet (2.6-7.1mg/L) compared to outlet (2.5-7.3mg/L). Low dissolved oxygen at the inlet is due to sewage getting into the tank. The higher dissolved oxygen during July'97 were due to sampling time (done at noon) when photosynthetic activity by the phytoplankton is maximum (releasing oxygen). The Biological Oxygen Demand observed at inlet, centre and outlet were 22.5 ± 5.8 mg/L, 20.0 ± 4.8 mg/L and 20.6 ± 5.2 mg/L respectively. The BOD at the inlet was understandably high, due to sewage entering into the tank at that point. The Chemical Oemand Demand values of the tank ranged from a low value of 56.0 mg/L during Oct'97 due to rains and to an high of 386.0 mg/L during Mar'97 at inlet, 58.3 mg/L to an high of 348 mg/L at Centre and 41.0 to 362.0 mg/L towards outlet. The higher values noticed during the Feb - Mar'97 months could be due to the sewage entering at sampling time and increased chemical concentration due to reduced volume of water during summer.

The various cat ions analysed showed higher values at all the points within the tank. The values of Calcium ranged from 68.9 to 248.0 mg/L at inlet, 73.2 to 160.0 mg/L at Centre and 60.6 to 244.0 mg/L at outlet. Such high values could be attributed to the domestic sewage that has detergents in it. The high values of Sodium ranging from 92 to 176 mg/L were observed at different points in the lake.

e) ULSOOR TANK:

Ulsoor tank, situated in the Eastern part of the city, spreads over an area of about 50 hectares. The tank receives direct industrial and domestic effluents from the surrounding areas of Tannery road, Ulsoor, etc. It has a park in its vicinity, a corporation swimming pool adjacent to the tank and a boat club provided by Karnataka State Tourism Development Corporation (KSTDC) for recreational purpose.

The colour of the water is greenish, with objectionable (fishy) odour. The temperature of the water during sampling periods ranged from 22 - 31°C with low transparency (4.5-16 Cms) and high turbidity (68-290 NTU).

The pH of the water samples were found mostly towards the alkaline ranging from 7.5-11.0. The high pH observed might be due to high planktonic activity, which makes use of the available carbon-di-oxide rendering the water alkaline and may be due to sewage. The Electrical Conductivity values were noticed to range from 0.6 - 1.2 ms/cm. The high values of EC were mostly due to higher dissolved solids. Total solids ranged between 460 - 884 mg/L and the Suspended Solids was about 200 mg/L at all sampling points in the lake during the study period. The high values of suspended solids are a result of high plankton density and suspended solids. The dissolved solids ranged from 246 - 644 mg/L indicating high dissolved solids. Dissolved Oxygen content was found to be 6.9 (±1.2) mg/L at inlet, 9.1 (±1.0) mg/L at Centre and 9.0 (±1.2) mg/L at outlet. High dissolved oxygen content of tank indicates high plankton activity, at the time of sampling (10-12 A.M). The Biological Oxygen Demand of the tank averaged at 22.6 mg/L. The Chemical Oxygen Demand values were found to be 231.4 mg/L, 216 mg/L and 221.3mg/L at the inlet, Centre and outlet respectively. The higher values of COD are a result of pollution from both point and non-point source pollution.

The study showed high concentrations of Chlorides at 131.4 mg/L at the inlet, 108.0 mg/L towards the Centre and 113.0 mg/L at outlet clearly indicating pollution due to high organic wastes The various cat ions analysed showed higher values at all points in the lake. Calcium showed

86.9 ± 32.9 mg/L, 89.5 ± 33.5 mg/L and 86.1 ± 40.7 mg/L at the inlet, towards Centre and outlet respectively. High values of Sodium ranging from 66 - 160 mg/L shows, pollution is mostly due to of domestic sewage.

f) YEDIUR TANK:

The Yediur tank is situated on the Kanakapura road in Jayanagar area of the south of the city covering an area of about four hectare. The tank has park and residential layout adjacent the tank. It was noticed that the tank receives both industrial and domestic sewage apart from the solid wastes dumped across the periphery of the tank serving as a breeding ground for mosquitoes and emiting obnoxious odour. This tank is heavily infested with microcystis which indicates the tank is polluted. The tank has two major inlets and two outlets.

The tank water was greenish owing to the high plankton density. High values of turbidity were noticed mainly due to plankton and sewage. Transparency of 5-14 cms indicates low light penetration. The temperature of the water measured during sampling time (10-11 am) varied from 23 - 29 °C.

The pH of the sample was mostly towards alkaline ranging from 7.5 to 10.1. The decrease in pH during the monsoons may be due to characteristic of sewage, decreased photosynthetic activity and also by the inflow of surface runoff waters. Maximum values noticed during summer months may be due to increased photosynthetic activity by the algal blooms.

The Dissolved Oxygen of the tank ranged from 4.0 to 10.0 mg/L at the Centre and from 3.8 to 8.9 mg/L towards the inlet. Relatively lower values at the inlet was due to the sewage and solid wastes preventing air-water interaction and decomposition of organic matter leading to lower dissolved oxygen. The higher values noticed at the Centre may be due to the higher planktonic density resulting in higher photosynthetic activity. The Chemical Oxygen

Demand values ranged from 84 mg/L in Oct'97 to a high of 378 mg/L during Apr'97 at the Centre and 112 mg/L in Sept'97 to high of 370 mg/L during Apr'97 towards inlet. During April'97 high values of COD was noticed, which may be due to less volume of water (evaporation) and continued inflow of sewage. The lower values during Sept-Oct'97 is due to inflow of catchments runoff resulted in dilution (Monsoon).The Biological Oxygen Demand values ranged from 14 - 32 mg/L towards the Centre of the lake and 17 - 31 mg/L towards the inlet where there was high influx of pollutants. The Suspended Solids in the lake was about 151.8 (avg) ± 58.6 (Sd) mg/L towards the Centre and 167.5 (avg) ±48.2 (Sd) mg/L towards the inlet. The high suspended solids were noticed during summer which may due to the algal blooms resulting in higher plankton density towards the Centre and due to sewage at the inlet. Maximum Total Solids were noticed both at inlet and towards the Centre which may be due to decreased water depth and inflow of sewage. The Total Dissolved Solids showed higher values towards the inlet ranging from 208 - 428 mg/L at an average of 272.0 mg/L. Similarly at the Centre it ranged from 212 to 402 mg/L at an average of 296.4 mg/L. The dissolved solids were noticed to be more during the summer at both points, which may due to the lower water levels.

The higher concentration of Chlorides, an indicator of organic pollution In the present study chlorides were noted at an average of 109.8 mg/L at the Centre and 96.0 mg/L towards the inlet. The Total Hardness ranged from 157.1 ± 30.5 mg/L towards the Centre to 146.5 ± 34.1 mg/L at inlet respectively. The main source of hardness in this lake was noticed which is due to the domestic and the industrial sewage apart from the non-point source runoff. The major cat ions Calcium, Magnesium, Potassium and Sodium showed noticeable variations. Calcium, Magnesium and Sodium were at 74.2 ± 19.5, 20.2 ± 10.9 and 80.1 ± 12.6 mg/L respectively.

g) KAMAKSHIPALYA TANK:

The Kamakshipalya tank situated on the western part of the city covers a small area of about an hectare. The tank is encroached on all the sides by slums with numerous small-scale industries located in its vicinity manufacturing plastic, chromium plating, etc. The tank once a source of drinking water (till the late 80's) receives direct effluent from both industries and the surrounding residential areas of Basaveshawara nagar, Saligrama, Kamakshipalya, etc.

The colour of the water was blackish, with high turbidity values ranging from 28 - 362 NTU and obnoxious odour throughout the study period.

The pH of the lake during the study period was acidic, ranging from 6.5 - 7.5. This could be due to the decay and decomposition of the accumulated organic matter and from the industrial sources. The Electrical Conductivity ranged from 1.27 - 2.09 ms/cm, indicating high amount of dissolved solids mostly from pollution. The Total Dissolved Solids of the water body was found to be 710.3 ± 114.2 mg/L at the point behind slum and 843.3 ± 179.2 mg/L towards the outlet. Higher values of Suspended Solids were noticed during the study period ranging from 108 mg/L to 410 mg/L which is due to influx of sewage. High amount of Suspended Solids leads to depletion in dissolved oxygen (especially if it is organic) apart from imparting high turbidity.

The low Dissolved Oxygen content of the lake indicates increased biological activity mainly due to organic pollution with values ranging from 0.5 mg/L to 3.9 mg/L reflecting the septic condition of the tank. The Chemical Oxygen Demand values ranged from 170 mg/L to an high of 621 mg/L. High values were observed during most of our study period (over 300mg/L) indicating severe chemical pollution due to sewage load. The Biological Oxygen Demand ranged from 27 mg/L to an high of 192 mg/L. Higher BOD values were noticed in samples collected behind slums (inlet) and could also be due to the dumping of solids composing organic wastes. The Chloride values of samples were found to be between 166.4 ± 76.898mg/L behind the slum and 221.7 ± 67.1mg/L at the outlet. Higher Sodium concentration ranging from 149 ± 73.2 mg/L suggests clear pollution by domestic sewage and high Calcium ranging from 57.2 to 192.0 mg/L could be due to the detergents from both domestic and industrial origin

Waste Management:

Waste management, a realistic appraisal of the health and hygienic condition is absolutely essential to understand the spillover effect on the neighboring localities. Apart from hygiene another variable which has an effect on environment is management of waste. Lot of waste is generated due to certain activates undertaken by slum people. Wastage generated due to household rotten activities, wastage generated due to business, commercial, industrial activities in the vicinity of the slum and bio-medical waste generated from places like primary health Centres, nursing homes and private clinics, all these things ultimately leads to generation of huge waste. This has posed severe challenges in the form of health hazards; breeding up of mosquitoes, stagnation of drainage water and contamination of soil, both surface and ground water.

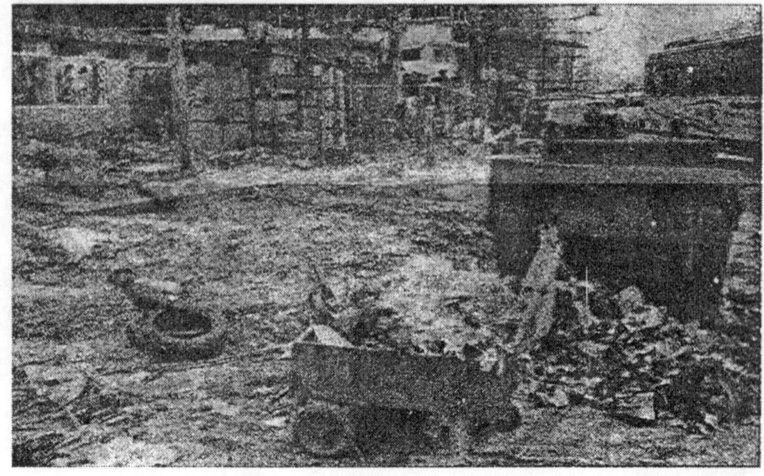

Figure - 4

The figures 3, 4 and 5 present the sorry state of solid waste management in the city in general and in and around slums in particular. One can see the garbage dumped haphazardly on the road side, spread all along the road blocking the so called foot paths including the road as such. This not only makes the pedestrians struggle for smooth walking but also makes the movement of vehicles troublesome. It also poses a great threat to the cleanliness of the city. It paves way for a number of contagious diseases creating health hazards among the public, particularly those who live in the vicinity and are more vulnerable to health risks. The figures throw light on one more aspect too that is the encroached foot paths and delayed repair works being stopped in between. The stones and mud dumped on the sides add up to the misery of the people making it horrible to walk through during rainy season.

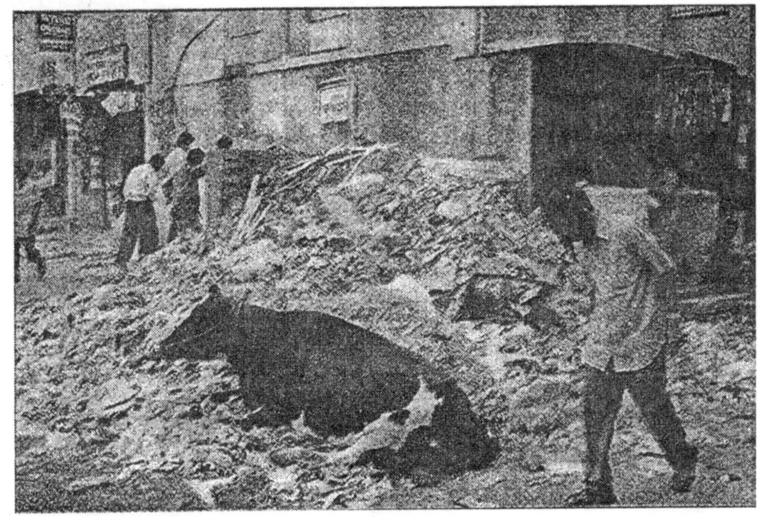

Figure - 5

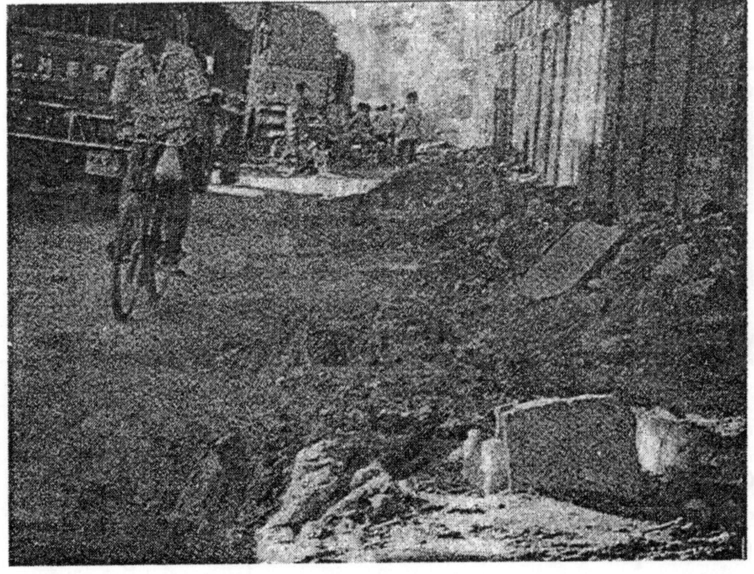

Figure - 6

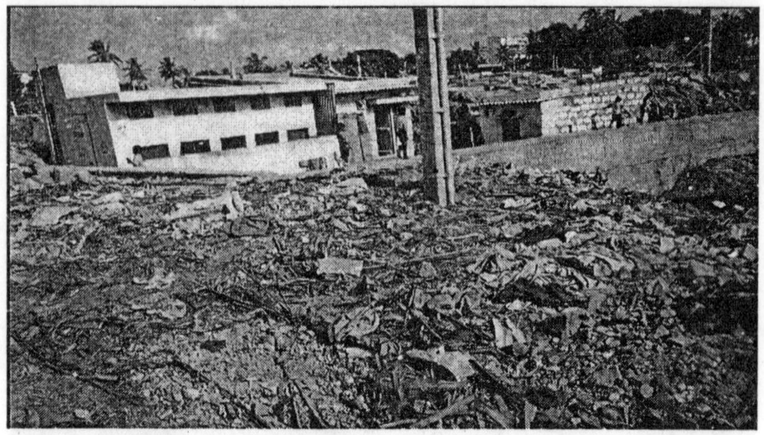

Figure - 7

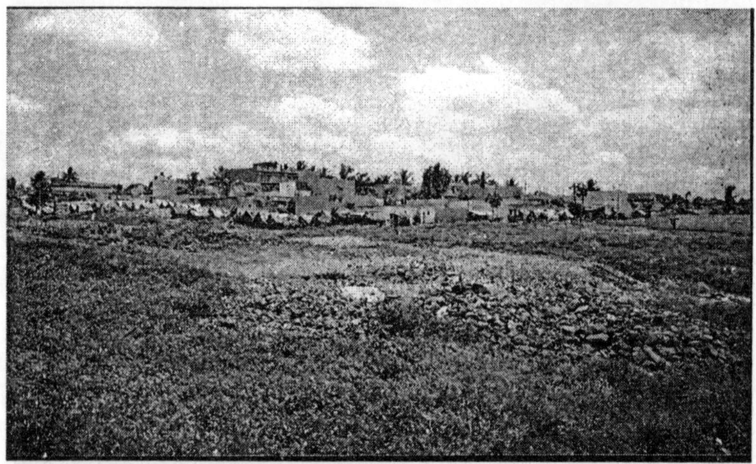

Figure - 8

Garbage and filth dumped in open space. This unfolds the story of garbage disposal in the city. All that is collected from the posh and hi-tech areas of the city are being dumped in the open space available near the slums making them uglier and unclean. This also reveals the importance given to the slums and their cleanliness.

Pollution due to unscientific handling and disposal of Bio-medical waste from all types of Health Care Establishments (HCE) like Hospital/Nursing Homes/Clinics/Dispensaries/Pathological Labs/Blood Banks, etc. has reached alarming rate in almost all cities/towns of our nation. In which Karnataka State is also one of the major contributor in providing Health Care facilities to public. The problem is more felt by the people residing at all major cities/towns in the state, particularly in the city of Bangalore with crowded population of more than thirty lakhs and having density of nearly five thousand HCE wide spread all over the districts. The emission and unscientific disposal of Bio-Medical Waste from all HCE has further worsened the situation. The release and disposal of Human Anatomical Waste, Microbiological Waste, Animal Waste, Waste Sharps like needles, syringes, discarded medicines and drugs, Solid waste like dressings, bedding, plaster, I.V. tubes, etc. Liquid waste like Blood and Body fluids, etc. into the atmosphere pollutes the surrounding air, water and soil. Because the Bio-Medical Waste consists of infectious microbial activity, it needs urgent/immediate attention of every occupier of Health Care Establishments and the general public in treatment and scientific disposal of Hazards Bio-Medical Waste.

The emission and disposal of liquid/solid waste from Hospitals/Nursing Homes, etc. contain most dangerous infection causing, spreading organisms/microbes which can cause/spread dreaded diseases like AIDS/Hepatitis/TB/Cancer/Cholera/Malaria/ Skin Diseases, etc. costing your life in one shot. (Brochures from pollution control board)

Researching recently for an article on e-waste was like seeing a horror movie. When burnt in illegal recycling junkyards, computers breathe black fumes of mercury, arsenic, lead, and other poisonous toxins. They become monsters of our techno-industrial growth. India, according to the New Delhi-based Toxic Links, annually generates about $1.5 billion worth of e-waste. An unofficial, unmonitored recycling industry in cities like New Delhi, Mumbai, and Chennai cannibalizes the electronic junk to salvage re-saleable metal. In the process, workers who handle the waste without protective clothing and the neighbourhood have their lungs, kidneys, nervous system, hearts, land and drinking water fatally ruined. E-waste refers to discarded electronics including computers, printers, mobile phones and other such hardware. Bangalore by itself is said to annually generate nearly 6000 tonnes of it. The Swiss are among few people in the world with know-how to safely dispose of it. Similarly, another horror story unfolds on our urban roads. (Lethal wastes: The Economic Times, 25 April 2004)

A recent study by the Chittaranjan National Cancer Institute, Kolkata, found that people in Delhi are about twice as likely to suffer from lung ailments as those in the countryside. While traffic pollution is the main cause, doctors say the smelting electronic parts at factories on the city's edges should not be discounted. Environmentalists also fear a critical contamination of soil and ground water from discarded ash and plastic residues.

Recyclers, many of them women and children, melt computer parts with acids, releasing a smoky stream of lead, dioxin and other toxins. Workers are "bound to inhale lead fumes," says Kishore Wankhade of Toxics Link, a group monitoring the handling of electronic waste. (E-waste a health hazard: The Indian Express, 11 April 2004)

Computer equipment is a complicated assembly of more than 1,000 components, many of which are hazardous and toxic. A major culprit in the hazardous waste areas is the computer monitor and television cathode ray tube (CRT), which contains five to eight pounds of lead. The non-biodegradable refuse from e-waste and other sources often ends up in land-fills or incinerators where toxic substances like residues of lead, cadmium, lethal mercury, carcinogenic asbestos, tin plates, arsenic, PVC and plastic waste, lead and cadmium batteries etc. contaminate the land, water and air, posing serious health hazards and affecting the environment. (PC waste leaves toxic taste: The Tribune, 22 March 2004)

According to a report released by NGO Toxics Link last week, a large amount of highly toxic e-waste is either illegally imported into the country or generated by business houses. The scrap contains a variety of heavy metals and other toxic compounds such as lead, mercury, arsenic, cadmium and brominated flame retardants. "A large amount of the e-waste we have discovered is being imported into country because it is cheaper to recycle it here. In the US it costs companies approximately $20 to recycle one computer. Instead, they make a profit by selling the scrap to an Indian trader for $5," explains environment activist and Toxics Link director Ravi Agrawal. (Toxic waste: Junkyards rip PCs to last bargaining chip: The Indian Express, 21 March 2004)

Electronic waste is piling up. How much, nobody knows. So, the government will conduct rapid assessment studies in cities like Bangalore, Kolkata and Chennai and set up a group to evolve a policy for this mounting problem. On the sidelines of a national meet on e-waste management Monday, Central Pollution Control Board chief V Rajagopalan said these studies could take six months or more. The group planned would, he said, involve the different stakeholders-government, industry, recyclers. (Government steps in as e-waste piles up: The Times of India, 16 March 2004)

Warning that the threat of e-waste was not limited to Delhi alone, a study "E-Waste in Chennai: Time is Running Out" released here this past week points out that the issue is a national one as the practice of computer and electronic waste dumping and recycling under very hazardous conditions is rampant in Chennai and Mumbai as well. Conducted by the non-government organisation, Toxics Link, the report points out that even as the domestic generation of e-waste is likely to increase soon with the high rate of obsolesce of technology, the "illegal" import of e-waste from developed countries continues unabated. (Warning on e-waste threat: The Hindu, 16 March 2004)

There is some alarming news on e-waste, waste generated out of junked computers. A report released recently found that dumping and recycling of this hazardous waste is rampant in Chennai and Mumbai. And it is not just waste from within the country but imported waste that is flooding the recycling market. It's a matter of concern as e-waste contains over 1000 substances and chemicals, many of which are toxic and which may create problems for those exposed directly in recycling units and also for the environment. Though the exact quantum of this waste is not known, there are indicators that it is on the rise and India will be the prime destination in the coming years. (India destination for e-waste; The Indian Express, 15 March 2004)

A new study conducted by the University of Florida environmental engineers reveals that electronic-age gizmos ranging from cell-phones to computer mice often release enough lead in laboratory tests to be classified as harzardous waste under the federal EPA (Environmental Protection Agency) regulations. The findings could prompt the federal government or individual States to change the disposal rules for millions of tones of electronic devices. More than 20 million personal computers became obsolete in 1998 alone, and more than 60 million personal computers are projected to meet the same fate in 2005, Townsend said. In research that began late in 2001, Townsend and four University of Florida graduate students examined cell-phones, printers, flat-panel monitors, keyboards, computer mice, remote controls, VCRs, laptops and central processing units, or CPUs. The e-devices were subjected to a standard EPA testing procedure for hazardous waste called the Toxicity Characteristic Leaching Procedure. It involves mixing the ground-up devices with an acid solution designed to simulate potential conditions in landfills. The mixture is rotated for 18 hours in a drum container, and the results are tested for eight hazardous metals: mercury, arsenic, cadmium, barium, silver, selenium, chromium and lead. (E-devices are environmental hazards: The Hindu Business Line, 4 March 2004)

There's worse new on the pollution front. The grey-eyed monster has incorporated another avatar in its arsenal: waste generated by electronic materials. The harsh reality is that Delhi is fast emerging as a centre for e-pollution. A recent report published by Toxics Link, an NGO, shows that the e-waste being dumped in the city spells imminent danger for the environment and human lives. 'E-waste comprises a broad range of electronic devices ranging from large household appliances such as refrigerators and ACs to cell-phones, stereos and computers,' informs Kishore of Toxics Link, "These electronic equipment contain substances which are toxic, such as lead and cadmium in circuit boards and mercury in switches and flat-screen monitors. Of the nearly 5 million PCs in India, 1.38 million are estimated to be outdated and could soon be added to the waste stream. 'Cyber-laws relating to the environment are as good as non-existent. This makes it tough to control the situation," says cyber law expert Pavan Duggal, "There are laws dealing with computers and networking, but there is a silence on how to scientifically eliminate obsolete machines." (E-waste: Pollution's latest dirty word: The Times of India, 6 January 2004)

12th December 2003 - *Mountains of e-waste - discarded parts of computers, mobile phones and other consumer electronics equipment - are quietly creating a new environmental problem in India.*

Thirty million computers are thrown out every year in the US alone, and many are dumped in India and China. Up to 70 per cent of the heavy metals in landfills come from electrical equipment waste. Now concerns are being raised on the impact the dumping - particularly evident in India's computer heartland, Delhi - is having on both the country's environment, and its people. "The problem is that these computers, which are quite old, have a lot of toxic material in them," Ravi Agraval, leader of campaign group Toxic Links, told BBC World Service's One Planet programme. "They have things like mercury, lead, flame retardants, and PVC-coated copper wire when you try and extract or recondition these computers you release these heavy metals and these chemicals. These are disasters for the environment."

E-waste heads to India, China and Bangladesh because computer "recycling" is a good business, with much money to be made. Computer recycling involves employing people to strip down the computers and extract parts that can be used again in machines to be sold on the high street. The rest is then burned or dumped, both of which are potentially highly hazardous to the environment. "The process of extraction uses all kinds of chemicals, like acids - which then get dumped into the soil and go into the groundwater," Mr Agraval said. "When you burn things like PVC-covered copper wire, you have emissions of very toxic chemicals like dioxins, which get released into the local environment." There are also fears that the recycling process, an unregulated industry in India, is also very harmful to the health of those employed to do it. In particular, the job involves exposure to a number of toxic chemicals both as part of the recycling process and within the computers themselves. "The people actually doing the brunt of the recycling are people on less than half a dollar a day - women and children working in very shanty-like, disastrous, inhuman conditions," Mr Agraval said. "When you burn things like PVC-covered copper wire, you have emissions of very toxic chemicals like dioxins, which get released into the local environment." There are also fears that the recycling process, an unregulated industry in India, is also very harmful to the health of those employed to do it. In particular, the job involves exposure to a number of toxic chemicals both as part of the recycling process and within the computers themselves. "The people actually doing the brunt of the recycling are people on less than half a dollar a day - women and children working in very shanty-like, disastrous, inhuman conditions," Mr Agraval said. "For them, it's the difference between poison and a livelihood." He added that a health survey had shown that recyclers regularly suffered from complaints such as respiratory diseases and skin rashes. "It's difficult to say when you're in that state of poverty what really affects what, but certainly they are people on the edge, and any such exposure can't be doing them any good."

Meanwhile in India, Mahinder Agowal, who represents the All Delhi Computer Traders Association, said that the risk to employees who recycled computers was relatively small. "Out of the 2,000 shops most are in a good condition, "he argued". Only some - very few - are in a bad condition. That happens in any market. "If you go to a cigarette shop you wouldn't expect it to be in a good condition, so I feel most of the shops are fine." However, one recycling shop visited by One Planet reporter Richard Hollingham - and credited by Mr Agowal's organisation - was clearly cramped with strong-smelling chemicals in the air. Mr Agowal defended his organisation's members, arguing that many of them had set up business with very little money. "Each will conduct business according to his own resources," he said. "We can't interfere with that."

As the personal computer, cell phones, and other electronic gadgets become an intrinsic part of modern life, evironmentalists around the globe are facing yet another development hazard - electrical and electronic waste, popularly known as 'e-waste' "Out of the 2,000 shops most are in a good condition," he argued. Only some - very few - are in a bad condition. That happens in any market.

"If you go to a cigarette shop you wouldn't expect it to be in a good condition, so I feel most of the shops are fine." However, one recycling shop visited by One Planet reporter Richard Hollingham - and credited by Mr Agowal's organisation - was clearly cramped with strong-smelling chemicals in the air. Mr Agowal defended his organisation's members, arguing that many of them had set up business with very little money. "Each will conduct business according to his own resources," he said. "We can't interfere with that."

'E-waste' is a collective name for discarded electronics devices that enter the stream from various sources. It includes electronic appliances such as televisions, personal computers, telephones, air conditioners, cell phones, electronic toys, etc. The list of e-waste is very large and can be further widened if one includes other electronic waste emanating from electrical appliances such as lifts, refrigerators, washing machines, dryers, and kitchen utilities, or even airplanes. Driven primarily by faster technological innovation and consequently a high rate of obsoleteness, this catalogue of new wastes poses a direct challenge, for its proper disposal or recycling in the present set up is expensive and technical. The issue has assumed serious global dimensions; e-waste creates serious worker, community and environmental problems, not only in production but also at the waste end (Toxics Link, 2003).

What concerns environmentalists is the growing market for the waste thus generated. A number of Asian countries are generally considered to be the main importers of e-wastes generated around the world. Importing countries can earn significant incomes from refurbishing used PCs and disassembling obsolete PCs, monitors, and circuit boards and then recovering gold, copper and other precious metals. Apart from metals, the equipment also contains highly sophisticated blends of metals, plastics, and other materials. The presence of hazardous substances such as lead, cadmium, and mercury in this e-waste makes working conditions dangerous.

Due to the hazards involved, disposing and recycling e-waste has serious legal and environmental implications. When computer waste is land filled or incinerated, it poses significant contamination problems. Landfills leach toxins into groundwater and incinerators emit toxic air pollutants including dioxins. Likewise, the recycling of computers has serious occupational and environmental implications, particularly when the recycling industry is often marginally profitable at best and often cannot afford to take the necessary precautions to protect the environment and worker health. (Toxics Link, 2003, scrapping the hi-tech myth - Computer waste in India. BAN and SVTC. 2002, Exporting Harm: The High-Tech Trashing of Asia)

References

1. *Census Reports,* 2001
2. Chakravarti, S. 1998: Deals on wheels *India Today,* Jan. 19.
3. Chakrabarthi, T. 1993: *Legality of Hazardous Waste Management in India,* Journal of Indian Association for Environmental Management. Vol, 20, P, 1-3, 1993.
4. Jha, U.C., 2004: Perspectives Environmental Issues and SAARC Economic and Political Weekly, April 24, 2004.pp, 1666, 1667 and 1668.
5. Karnataka State Slum Clearance Board - Details of Total Slums and Declared Slums in Bangalore City.
6. Mehra, A., M.E. Farago, D.K. Banerjee 1998: Impact of fly ash from coal-fired power stations in Delhi, with particular reference to metal contamination. *Environment Monitoring Assessment* 50 (1):1535.

7. Mostardi, R.A., D. Leonard 1974: Air pollution and cardiopulmonary function. *Arch. Environ. Health* 29:32528.
8. Ghosh , Rekha, D.S. Chatterjee, 2004: Environmental Geology, Geo-ecosystem Protection in Mining Areas, Capital Publishing Company, New Delhi.
9. Shah, J., T. -Nagpal. eds. 1997: *Urban Air Quality Management Strategy in Asia (URBAIR). Greater Mumbai Reports. World Bank Tech. Pap. No. 381,* World Bank, Washington, DC.
10. Smith, K.R., Y. -Liu 1994: *Indoor air pollution in developing countries in The Epidemiology of Lung Cancer,* ed. J Samet, pp. 15184. New York: Marcel Dekker.
11. US Environmental Protection Agency. 1982: *Review of the National Ambient Air Quality Standard for Particulate Matter: Assessment of Scientific and Technical Information*. Research Triangle Park, NC: US EPA.

CHAPTER III

SLUM SCENE– A HISTORICAL PERSPECTIVE

Slum Scene – A Historical Perspective

Urbanisation and slums have been a subject matter of a wide-range of sociological and anthropological studies though a great deal of research material is now available in series of volumes brought out by the Indian Council of Social Science Research.

Yet an attempt has been made here to make a critical review of some studies which throw some light on the nature of interconnection across Urbanisation, slums and environmental degradation.

Sociologists in the west have made attempts to study the nature of slums and their pattern of growth in different social contexts. Some of the most popular theories regarding slums are E.W.Burge's theory of changes in urban land use patterns; Homer Hoytls' Sector theory; Herbert Gans' Typology of the slums. Herbert Gans in his book; *Urban Villages,* discusses about two types of slums. They are what he calls, "Entry area" that is the area inhabited by whom he calls "social rejects". In the "entry area" newcomers to the city find their first place to live in. Here they try to adopt their non-urban institutions and cultures to the urban milieu. In the second type low rent neighbourhood, those people who have not succeeded and are not going to succeed are predominant. This he calls 'urban jungle', such a clear-cut dichotomy of slums though theoretically appear to be very attractive empirically is extremely difficult to observe particularly in Indian cities. People migrating from rural areas settle in urban areas according to their caste and regional affinities. A majority of the slum dwellers are poor and provide shelter to criminals and prostitutes.

Another aspect of slums is ecological consequences of growth of slums and the phenomenal increase in slum population. Like other human beings slum people meddle too much with environment in which they live. Forced to eke out their bread they engage themselves in a wide variety of activities which directly impinge on the environment ultimately rapidly leading to the degradation, demoralisation, and disempowerment of slum people. Pushed to hand–to-mouth existence, they seem neither have any knowledge, awareness of the wide range of adverse implications that their lifestyles and the living conditions have for the welfare, well being of not only themselves but also of other people who might live in the vicinity of slums. Given the physical proximity of the slums with main stream urban settlement, the grave-health –risks which urban people might get exposed to and become increasingly vulnerable cannot however be ignored. One such study which touch upon this problem in the one undertaken by Ratana Naidu.

It is not difficult to recognise ecological consequences of growth of slums even though it received a scant attention. Ratana Naidu observed in her study of slums in Hyderabad and Secundrabad that in the poorer countries infrastructural facilities like transportation and communication, schools, shops, hospitals and sanitary conditions remain low and continues to remain inadequate in spite of accelerated growth of the city peripheries. The middle and upper classes stay near the centre of business district and land values around these areas remain perhaps the highest in the metropolis. She also observed that though some slums developed near the business district, most of the slums developed around the industries and other major commercial and business establishments. This establishment releases a wider range of pollutants into the atmosphere.

There are theories, which provide valuable insights into the dynamics of urban life situation of urbanites in general and slum people in particular, though these theories cannot be blindly applied to situations that obtain in urban India. Of all the theories, the theory of 'culture of poverty' by Oscar Lewis deserves special mention. It makes a serious examination of the nature of impact that slums could cause on urban life. Why slums are regarded as purveyors of pollution of life in towns and cities? Answer lies in the way slum people live their life. Theory of culture of poverty, seen in detail, has the following features: - Lack of effective participation and integration of the slum people in the major institutions of the large society; low wages; chronic unemployment; poor housing conditions; low level organisation; At the family level the absence of childhood as a specially prolonged and protected stage in the life cycle leading to early initiation into sex, free unions or consensual marriages. At the level of individual, major characteristics are strong feelings of marginality, helplessness, dependency and inferiority, etc. Given this culture, slum people have become increasingly vulnerable to grave-health risks including sexually transmitted diseases and through them they could spread across urban people.

The theories of culture of poverty have become a subject matter of great deal of discussion. Hyman Rodman in his study of the lower class families entitled, *The culture of poverty in Trinidad* opines that culture and personality of member of the lower class are not altogether determined by the circumstances of lower class life.

Review of literature on slums makes one thing clear; that slums have been predominantly viewed as social-disorganisations. One of the most persistent reasons for the unabated growth of slums which started spreading to medium towns and small towns is rural urban migration, which is in turn caused by factors called 'push factors' operating in the village like high unemployment, lack of resources primarily land other agricultural inputs and poverty forced villagers to move over to towns and cities almost invariably in search of source of earning their livelihood. The patterns of settlement of migrants increasingly depend upon and determined by caste, language, regional and kinship affiliations. Land value depends upon the land use patterns. Around the industrial and commercial activities the land value increase and vice versa. Slum people are bound to be poor because of the peculiar factors associated with the culture, which they inherit across generations and generations, while all these things are fairly well known, what has been less known, not sufficiently recognised is the adverse environmental changes that inevitably follow the growth of slums and slum people. Environmental degradation has been taking place increasingly due to pollution of air, water, soil and noise and this has certainly posed grave health risks not speak of the steady deterioration taking place in the quality and productivity of environmental resources. This has been sufficiently recognised so repeatedly recognised that it has become a self-evident truth. It is indeed surprising that slum population primarily by their life styles and conditions of living could equally spoil the environment and this has gone unrecognised. The present study takes a point of departure in that it seeks to analyze the adverse effects that slums can produce on urban environment and the impact of urban environment on slum population. This aspect of slum has remained neglected in the field of Sociology of slums. The present study patently seeks to fill this gap in our knowledge and understanding of slums (M. S. Dhadve, 1988).

Family relations in slums are another important and interesting feature. In the context of slum population some of the investigations carried out into fertility behaviour have indicated that with the rise in Socio-Economic status, the number of children desired also increased. The responses of Women in Calcutta show that under existing conditions they would prefer two children, while under 'Ideal' condition they would prefer four (J.B. Mukherjee, 1961). In contrast to this, Raman has referred to the findings of D.N.Majumdar (1960) in Kanpur and C. Chandrashekaran (1961) in Mysore. In Kanpur, no difference was found in the number of children desired by illiterate and primary educated women, but the number desired was less in the case of secondary and college educated women. In Bangalore city, high educational level and high economic status were found to be correlated with desire to have a small family.

Increase in the size of family and poverty are differentially correlated in different socio-economic context. In the context of slums increase in the number of children, with lack of spacing in the birth of children lead to high maternal mortality rates, low weight of new born children, mal nutrition, and Urbanisation so on and so forth. Such children when they grow up somehow or the other not only become drain resources but also become purveyors of dirt, disease, squalor, increasing juvenile criminal behaviour. Having exposed to violent disorganised social life both at home as well as outside they become the potential offenders, budding criminals, drug peddlers. Given their pathological life style, the adverse impact of their life style on environment is unimaginable. Some of these things will be discussed with reference to empirical data in the following chapters.

T.G. Megee, points out: "in fact the squatter settlements and slums of South-east Asian cities are the symptoms of much wider problems in societies of South-east Asia, problems for which the piecemeal provision of housing can be little more than palliative measure; majority of the South-east Asian nations tend to evolve policies of economic development in order promote balance in the flow of investment and people between rural and urban societies (M. S. Dhadve, 1988).

Net effect of this is number of slums is increasing and multiplying. Growth of slums is by no means confined to big cities. They have spread very fast to small and medium towns as well. Clinard aptly describes nature of slums; inadequate housing, deficient facilities, over-crowding and congestion characterize a slum. Further he says slum people develop their own culture which is a sub-culture with a set of norms and values which is reflected in poor sanitation and health practices, deviant Behaviour, characteristic attributes of apathy and social isolation. A slum is isolated from the mainstream society and regarded as inferior and looked at by the outside world suspiciously.

Shelters around drainages, government vacant sites, work sites and other abandoned regions in the city spring up both as cause and consequences of uneven and unplanned urban growth and have come to pose environmental threats. What is however not taken serious note of by administrators, town planners and researchers is the environmental degradation that follows the proliferation of slums. Slums in urban areas produce a serious effect; that is the adverse environmental changes that accompany rather tenaciously the process of Urbanisation that inevitably follow the growth of slums and slum people. Environmental degradation has been taking place increasingly due to unprecedented pressure on infrastructure and due to rapid growth of urban population. Depletion of renewable and non-renewable resources, population pressure, and unabated generation of solid waste: bio-medical waste, municipal waste and liquid waste to mention a few resulted in the pollution of water, air, soil and noise. This posed grave-risks and the quality and productivity of people have suffered. This has been sufficiently recognised and recorded by wide array of research studies. It is indeed sad to note that slum population primarily by their life style and conditions of living could equally spoil the environment. The present study takes a point of departure in that it seeks to analyze the adverse effects that slums can produce on urban population and urban environment. This constitutes the crux of the study. The present study patently seeks to fill this gap in our knowledge and understanding of slums and the impact of the slums on urban environment. Reiterating this gap, attempt is made here to review the available literature on Urbanisation particularly as these studies high light the negative impact of slums on urban life. (M.S. Dhadve, 1988 pp.No. 39 to52)

The study on Diarrhea and Hygiene in Lucknow Slums under the aegis of Gomti River Pollution Control Project, supported by Department for International Development, Ankur along with London School of Hygiene & Tropical Medicine, U.K. conducted between January and July'1996.

The study, Diarrhea & Hygiene in Lucknow Slums, conducted in low income group pockets of Lucknow, aimed at identifying hygiene practices of the slum dwellers, which put them at risk of diarrheal incidences. People's beliefs and perceptions regarding diarrhea were also probed. Behavioural trials were conducted to work out the strategy to change the following risk practices.

Due to their size, physiology, and behaviour, children are more vulnerable than adults to environmental hazards. Children are more heavily exposed to toxins in proportion to their body weight, and have more years of life ahead of them in which they may suffer long-term effects from early exposure. Prenatal conditions, which can be influenced by environmental conditions, cause 20 *per cent* of deaths worldwide in children under age 5. Furthermore, fetal exposure to chemicals such as lead increases a child's chances of having brain damage or developmental problems. Typical childhood behaviours, such as crawling and putting objects in the mouth, can also lead to increased risks. Children between ages 5 and 18 may face higher risks of injuries, including exposure to hazardous chemicals, due to their growing participation in household chores and work outside of the home. Many school-age children attend schools without sanitation facilities, making them more likely to contract various diseases and less likely to go to school.

GROWTH OF SLUMS IN BANGALORE CITY

Rapid Growth of Urban Population

Urbanisation and urban growth will be one of the major challenges. The growing requirement of food will place enormous pressure on land resources. Farmers with small plots will be forced to 'mine' their land by cutting the remaining trees of young age in ecologically destructive practices of crop intensification on marginal land. The increased demand for fuel wood, which is the major source of household fuel among the low-income groups of the population, will lead to further deforestation. This would naturally be accompanied by the associated problem of widespread soil erosion, watershed damage and flooding. Urban areas are particularly prone to this problem, but rural areas are not entirely free from it either. The resultant health hazards include water-borne diseases, respiratory diseases, asthma (especially among the young and the aged) and an increased risk of cancer.

South Asian countries are likely to encounter many problems of food scarcity in this century. The production will fall short of requirements. According to estimates, India would need 400-500 million tones of food grains by 2050, and the other countries of the region would need about 200 million tones. By 2050 South Asia will need to produce around 650 million tones of food grains (*FAO Yearbook Production*, Rome 1998). India alone can technically produce enough food for the entire population of South Asia, but at an enormous economic cost and by placing a heavy burden on the environment and water. The storage of food in India, Pakistan, Bangladesh and Nepal, will put tremendous pressure on environmental resources. The environment in South Asia will come under increasing threat for several decades. The World Bank (1991) estimates that 60 per cent of the tropical forest area cleared for each year makes room for new agriculture settlements. Agricultural encroachment for forest area may take two paths: the gradual 'nibbling' at small islands of rain forests located within a vast area of cleared land; or the massive influx of settlers into previously inaccessible large areas of forest following logging operations or major infrastructure development projects. The first path is more typical in mountainous areas while the second occurs predominantly in lowlands. In highland areas, settlers creep up the slopes, clearing trees, and leading to soil erosion and downstream flooding during the monsoon and water shortage during the dry monsoon, as well as downstream siltation of rivers and dams. The latter type of encroachment will be more dominant in Nepal, Sri Lanka and the hilly regions of India, And in Plains, the soil will be burdened with excessive use of pesticides, insecticides and chemical manure. This will deteriorate the soil further, pollute water bodies and cause cascading effects on fisheries and marine animals.

In the past two decades the World's urban population has increased by about a billion from 1.35 to 2.28 billion. The bulk of this increase has been (about 60 per cent) in Asia and most of it in the South Asian countries. As per the estimates, urban population is close to 400 million in South Asia. This will increase to 800 million in 20 years. In most South Asian cities, urban infrastructure built slowly over several decades, is already under severe strain with continuous migration from rural areas, Indian society is no exception to this. Rural migrants in search of better living conditions in urban areas, remain below the acceptable threshold even though urban living conditions have improved over in the last 50 years since independence.

The cities will find it extremely difficult to cope with demands for civic services and basic infrastructure. Low income groups will create slums.

Table – No.1. URBAN AGGLOMERATION/CITIES HAVING POPULATION OF MORE THAN ONE MILLION IN INDIA - 2001

Rank in 2001	Urban Agglomeration/City (1,000,000+Population)	Population		
		Persons	Males	Females
1	Greater Mumbai	16368084	8979172	7388912
2	Kolkata	13216546	7072114	6144432
3	Delhi	12791458	7021896	5769562
4	Chennai	6424624	3294328	3130296
5	Bangalore	5686844	2983926	2702918
6	Hyderabad	5533640	2854938	2678702
7	Ahmadabad	4519278	2397728	2121550
8	Pune	3755525	1980941	1774584
9	Surat	2811466	1597093	1214373
10	Kanpur	2690486	1440140	1250346
11	Jaipur	2324319	1239711	1084608
12	Lucknow	2266933	1199273	1067660
13	Nagpur	2122965	1097723	1025242
14	Patna	1707429	925857	781572
15	Indore	1639044	861758	777286
16	Vadodara	1492398	783237	709161
17	Bhopal	1454830	766602	688228
18	Coimbatore	1446034	743161	702873
19	Ludhiana	1395053	789868	605185
20	Kochi	1355406	670462	684944
21	Visakhapatnam	1329472	674080	655392
22	Agra	1321410	708622	612788
23	Varanasi	1211749	644922	566827

24	Madurai	1194665	604728	589937
25	Meerut	1167399	624904	542495
26	Nashik	1152048	619962	532086
27	Jabalpur	1117200	588556	528644
28	Jamshedpur	1101804	580336	521468
29	Asansol	1090171	576813	513358
30	Dhanbad	1064357	578602	485755
31	Faridabad	1054981	580548	474433
32	Allahabad	1049579	581876	467703
33	Amritsar	1011327	543638	467689
34	Vijayawada	1011152	531084	480068
35	Rajkot	1002160	525797	476363
	TOTAL	**107881836**	**57664396**	**50217440**

Source: Directorate of Census Operation Paper II - 2001 Census.

Table –No. 2.URBAN AGGLOMERATION/ CITIES HAVING POPULATION OF OVER ONE MILLION

Census year	Number of urban Agglomeration/ cities	Population (Million)	per cent of population of urban	
			Total Population	Urban Population
1901	1	1.51	0.63	5.84
1911	2	2.79	1.11	10.76
1921	2	3.17	1.26	11.29
1931	2	3.45	1.24	10.32
1941	2	5.37	1.68	12.16
1951	5	12.00	3.32	19.22
1961	7	18.47	4.21	23.40
1971	9	28.48	5.20	26.10
1981@	12	43.33	6.34	27.48
1991+	23	71.00	8.39	32.63

Source: Office of Registrar General of India.

@ The 1981 census could not be held in Assam and the proportional figures

For 1981 for Assam have been worked out by inter-polation.

\+ The 1991 census was not held in J&K. The proportional figures include the projected population for J&K.

Table –No. 3

Rural – Urban distribution of population – India and states/Union territories: 2001

Table –No. 3Rural – Urban distribution of population – India and states/Union territories: 2001						
Sl. No	India/State / Union territory*	T/R/U	Population			*Per cent* urban population
			Persons	Males	Females	
1	2	3	5	6	7	8
	INDIA	T	1,027,015,247	531,277,078	495,738,169	27.78
		R	741,660,293	381,141,184	360,519,109	
		U	285,354,954	150,135,894	135,219,060	
	State/ Union territory*					
1	Jammu & Kashmir	T	10,069,917	5,300,574	4,769,343	24.88
		R	7,564,608	3,925,846	3,638,762	
		U	2,505,309	1,374,728	1,130,581	
2	Himachal Pradesh	T	6,077,248	3,085,256	2,991,992	9.79
		R	5,482,367	2,754,251	2,728,116	
		U	594,881	331,005	263,876	
3	Punjab	T	24,289,296	12,963,362	11,325,934	33.95
		R	16,043,730	8,500,647	7,543,083	
		U	8,245,566	4,462,715	3,782,851	
4	Chandigarh*	T	900,914	508,224	392,690	89.78
		R	92,118	56,837	35,281	
		U	808,796	451,387	357,409	

5	Uttaranchal	T	8,479,562	4,316,401	4,163,161	25.59
		R	6,309,317	3,143,380	3,165,937	
		U	2,170,245	1,173,021	997,224	
6	Haryana	T	21,082,989	11,327,658	9,755,331	29
		R	14,968,850	8,017,622	6,951,228	
		U	6,114,139	3,310,036	2,804,103	
7	Delhi*	T	13,782,976	7,570,890	6,212,086	93.01
		R	963,215	533,219	429,996	
		U	12,819,761	7,037,671	5,782,090	
8	Rajasthan	T	56,473,122	29,381,657	27,091,465	23.38
		R	43,267,678	22,394,479	20,873,199	
		U	13,205,444	6,987,178	6,218,266	
9	Uttar Pradesh	T	166,052,859	87,466,301	78,586,558	20.78
		R	131,540,230	69,096,765	62,443,465	
		U	34,512,629	18,369,536	16,143,093	
10	Bihar	T	82,878,796	43,153,964	39,724,832	10.47
		R	74,199,596	38,510,686	35,688,910	
		U	8,679,200	4,643,278	4,035,922	
11	Sikkim	T	540,493	288,217	252,276	11.1
		R	480,488	255,386	225,102	
		U	60,005	32,831	27,174	
12	Arunachal Pradesh	T	1,091,117	573,951	517,166	20.41
		R	868,429	453,560	414,869	
		U	222,688	120,391	102,297	
13	Nagaland	T	1,988,636	1,041,686	946,950	17.74
		R	1,635,815	846,651	789,164	
		U	352,821	195,035	157,786	
14	Manipur	T	2,388,634	1,207,338	1,181,296	23.88
		R	1,818,224	923,428	894,796	
		U	570,410	283,910	286,500	
15	Mizoram	T	891,058	459,783	431,275	49.5
		R	450,018	233,718	216,300	
		U	441,040	226,065	214,975	
16	Tripura	T	3,191,168	1,636,138	1,555,030	17.02
		R	2,648,074	1,359,288	1,288,786	
		U	543,094	276,850	266,244	
17	Meghalaya	T	2,306,069	1,167,840	1,138,229	19.63
		R	1,853,457	939,803	913,654	
		U	452,612	228,037	224,575	

18	Assam	T	26,638,407	13,787,799	12,850,608	12.72
		R	23,248,994	11,983,157	11,265,837	
		U	3,389,413	1,804,642	1,584,771	
19	West Bengal	T	80,221,171	41,487,694	38,733,477	28.03
		R	57,734,690	29,606,028	28,128,662	
		U	22,486,481	11,881,666	10,604,815	
20	Jharkhand	T	26,909,428	13,861,277	13,048,151	22.25
		R	20,922,731	10,660,430	10,262,301	
		U	5,986,697	3,200,847	2,785,850	
21	Orissa	T	36,706,920	18,612,340	18,094,580	14.97
		R	31,210,602	15,711,853	15,498,749	
		U	5,496,318	2,900,487	2,595,831	
22	Chhatisgarh	T	20,795,956	10,452,426	10,343,530	20.08
		R	16,620,627	8,290,983	8,329,644	
		U	4,175,329	2,161,443	2,013,886	
23	Madhya Pradesh	T	60,385,118	31,456,873	28,928,245	26.67
		R	44,282,528	22,975,256	21,307,272	
		U	16,102,590	8,481,617	7,620,973	
24	Gujarat	T	50,596,992	26,344,053	24,252,939	37.35
		R	31,697,615	16,289,423	15,408,192	
		U	18,899,377	10,054,630	8,844,747	
25	Daman & Diu*	T	158,059	92,478	65,581	36.26
		R	100,740	63,576	37,164	
		U	57,319	28,902	28,417	
26	Dadra & Nagar Haveli*	T	220,451	121,731	98,720	22.89
		R	169,995	91,887	78,108	
		U	50,456	29,844	20,612	
27	Maharashtra	T	96,752,247	50,334,270	46,417,977	42.4
		R	55,732,513	28,443,238	27,289,275	
		U	41,019,734	21,891,032	19,128,702	
28	Andhra Pradesh	T	75,727,541	38,286,811	37,440,730	27.08
		R	55,223,944	27,852,179	27,371,765	
		U	20,503,597	10,434,632	10,068,965	
29	Karnataka	T	52,733,958	26,856,343	25,877,615	33.98
		R	34,814,100	17,618,593	17,195,507	
		U	17,919,858	9,237,750	8,682,108	
30	Goa	T	1,343,998	685,617	658,381	49.77
		R	675,129	339,626	335,503	
		U	668,869	345,991	322,878	

31	Lakshadweep*	T	60,595	31,118	29,477	44.47
		R	33,647	17,196	16,451	
		U	26,948	13,922	13,026	
32	Kerala	T	31,838,619	15,468,664	16,369,955	25.97
		R	23,571,484	11,450,785	12,120,699	
		U	8,267,135	4,017,879	4,249,256	
33	Tamil Nadu	T	62,110,839	31,268,654	30,842,185	43.86
		R	34,869,286	17,508,985	17,360,301	
		U	27,241,553	13,759,669	13,481,884	
34	Pondicherry*	T	973,829	486,705	487,124	66.57
		R	325,596	163,586	162,010	
		U	648,233	323,119	325,114	
35	Andaman & Nicobar Islands*	T	356,265	192,985	163,280	32.67
		R	239,858	128,837	111,021	
		U	116,407	64,148	52,259	

Notes

1. The total, rural and urban population of India includes the estimated total, rural and urban population of entire Kachch district, Morvi, Maliya-Miyana and Wankaner taluks of Rajkot district, Jodiya taluka of Jamnagar district of Gujarat state and estimated total and rural population of entire Kinnaur district of Himanchal Pradesh where population enumeration of Census of India, 2001 could not be conducted due to natural calamities.

2 The figures of total, rural and urban population of Himachal Pradesh state have been arrived at after including the estimated total and rural population of entire Kinnaur district where population enumeration of Census of India, 2001 could not be conducted due to natural calamity.

3 The figures of total, rural and urban population of Gujarat state have been arrived at after including the estimated total, rural and urban population of entire Kachchh district, Morvi, Maliya-Miyana and Wankaner taluks of Rajkot district, Jodiya taluka of Jamnagar district

where population enumeration of the census of India, 2001 could not be conducted due to natural calamity.

Source: Census of India 2001.

Table – No. 4. Urban Agglomerations/Towns by Class/ Category: Census of India 2001:

Class	Population Size	No. of UAs /Towns
Class I	1,00,000 and above	393
Class II	50,000 - 99,999	401
Class III	20,000 - 49,999	1,151
Class IV	10,000 - 19,999	1,344
Class V	5,000 - 9,999	888
Class VI	Less than 5,000	191
Unclassified		10*
All classes		**4378**

Note: Data is provisional
Population Census 2001 could not be held in these towns/cities of Gujarat state on account of national calamity
Source: Office of the Registrar General of India. (Population totals for India & States for the Census of India – 2001)

Note: Data is provisionalPopulation Census 2001 could not be held in these towns/cities of Gujarat state on account of national calamity

Source: Office of the Registrar General of India. (Population totals for India & States for the Census of India – 2001)

Table –No. 5. Trends in Urbanisation in India , 1901-1991

Census Years	Total Population	Urban Population	No. of towns/ UAs	Per centage of Urban Population to Total Population	Decadal Urban Growth Rate	Annual Exponentia l Growth Rate	Annual Gain in Per centage of Urban Population	Annual Rate of Gain in Per centage of Urban Population
1901	238,396,327	25,854,967	1,827	10.85	NA	NA	NA	NA
1911	252,093,390	25,948,431	1,815	10.29	0.36	0.04	-0.06	-0.51
1921	251,321,213	28,091,299	1,949	11.18	8.26	0.8	0.09	0.86
1931	278,977,238	33,462,539	2,072	11.99	19.12	1.77	0.08	0.73
1941	318,660,580	44,162,191	2,250	13.86	31.98	2.81	0.19	1.55
1951	361,088,090	62,443,709	2,843	17.29	41.4	3.52	0.34	2.48
1961	439,234,771	78,936,603	2,365	17.97	26.41	2.37	0.07	0.39
1971	548,159,652	109,113,977	2,590	19.91	38.23	3.29	0.19	1.08
1981	683,329,097	159,462,547	3,301	23.34	46.14	3.87	0.34	1.72
1991	846,302,688	217,611,012	3,697	25.71	36.47	3.16	0.24	1.02

Note:

1. Includes the interpolated population of Assam for 1981; the total population is 18,041,248 and urban population is 1,782,376
2. Includes the projected population of Jammu & Kashmir for 1991; the total population is 7,718,700 and urban population 1,839,400
3. N.A; Not applicable

Source: Census of India , 1991, General Population Tables, Part II-A(i), Office of the Registrar General & Census, Commissioner, GOI, New Delhi

Table –No. 6. Identified/Estimated Slum Population of Million-Plus Cities, 1991 & 2001 (In million).

City	1991				2001 #		
	Total Populatio n	Slum Popu-lation		Per centage	Total Popu-lation	Slum Popu-lation	Per centage
Greater Bombay	12.6	4.32	*	34.3	17.07	5.86	34.3
Calcutta	11.02	3.63	*	32.93	13.11	4.31	32.9
Delhi	8.42	2.25		26.7	12.22	3.26	26.7
Madras	5.42	1.53		28.13	6.98	1.96	28.1
Hyderabad	4.34	0.86		19.78	6.3	1.25	19.8
Banga-lore	4.13	0.52		12.5	6.36	0.79	12.5
Ahmedaba d	3.31	0.67	*	20.23	4.36	0.89	20.31
Pune	2.49	0.41	*	16.44	3.53	0.58	16.3
Kanpur	2.03	0.42		20.55	2.49	0.51	20.6
Lucknow	1.67	0.28		16.64	2.26	0.37	16.6
Nagpur	1.66	0.53	*	31.85	2.32	0.74	31.9

Nagpur	1.66	0.53	*	31.85	2.32	0.74	31.9
Surat	1.52	0.39	*	25.67	2.29	0.58	25.4
Jaipur	1.52	0.44	*	28.98	2.21	0.64	29.1
Kochi	1.14	0.28	*	24.55	1.54	0.38	24.8
Vado-dara	1.13	0.21		18.31	1.71	0.31	18.3
Indore	1.11	0.17	*	15.33	1.54	0.23	15.2
Coim-batore	1.1	0.1		8.7	1.33	0.12	8.7
Patna	1.1	0.7	*	63.66	1.53	0.97	63.5
Madurai	1.09	0.2		17.99	1.31	0.24	18
Bhopal	1.06	0.15	*	14.11	1.53	0.21	13.99
Vishakhapatnam	1.06	0.27		25.2	1.67	0.42	25.2
Ludhiana	1.04	0.37		35.36	1.63	0.58	35.4
Varanasi	1.03	0.21		20.12	1.33	0.27	20.1
Total	**71**	**18.87**		**26.57**	**96.63**	**25.48**	**26.37**

Note:

1. Classification of the size of cities is based on 1991 census
2. Total is different because of rounding off the figures
3. * Based on the per centage identified slum population of 1981
4. # Estimated

Source: Central Statistical Organisation, Compendium of Environment Statistics, 1997, M/o, Planning & Programme Implementation, GOI, New Delhi

URBANISATION IN KARNATAKA:

The below table gives details regarding total number of urban agglomerations and towns from 1901 to 2001, growth of urban population in Karnataka, total population, urban population, decennial growth rate, etc. for Karnataka State for the Censuses of 1901 to 2001. This statement brings out the trends in Urbanisation since 1901.

It is seen from the statement that the proportion of urban population in the State has increased from 12.59 per cent in 1901 to an all time high of 33.98 per cent in 2001.

The decennial growth rate during 1941-51 has been the highest ever viz., 61.19 per cent. This is due to the increase in the number of towns from 213 in 1941 to 289 in 1951 and urban population as a consequence. Similarly the urban population recorded a growth rate of 50.65 per cent during 1971-81 due to a higher number of places classified as towns and also due to higher growth rates recorded by some of the towns. There is a fall in the decennial growth rate from 29.62 per cent in 1991 to 28-85 per cent in 2001 although acceleration of urban population during 1991-2001 is of higher order.

Table – No. 7. Trends in Urbanisation in Karnataka, 1901-2001

Census Year	Total number of UAs/ Towns	Total Population	Total urban population	*Per cent* urban population	Decennial growth		Annual exponential growth rate (urban)
					Absolute	*Per cent*	
1	2	3	4	5	6	7	*8*
1901	219	13,054,754	1,642,994	12.59	-	-	-
1911	184	13,525,251	1,570,570	11.61	-72,424	-4.41	-0.45
1921	198	13,377,599	1,845,819	13.80	+275,249	17.53	1.61
1931	216	14,632,992	2,245,684	15 35	+399,865	21.66	1.96
1941	213	16,255,368	2,762,861	17.00	+517,177	23.03	2.07
1951	289	19,401,956	4,453,480	22.95	+1,690,619	61.19	4.77
1961	231	23,586,772	5,266,493	22.33	+813,013	18.26	1.68
1971*	230	29,299,014	7,122,093	24.31	+1,855,600	35.23	3.02
1981*	250	37,135,714	10,729,606	28.89	+3,607,513	50.65	4.1
1991*	253	44,977,201	13,907,788	30.92	+3,178,182	29.62	2.59
2001*	237	52,733,958	17,919,858	33.98	+4,012,070	28.85	2.53

* The concept of urban agglomeration was introduced in 1971 Census. For the purpose of this statement an urban agglomeration with all its constituent units is reckoned as a single unit for all the censuses to present a comparative picture. The constituent units of the concerned urban agglomerations are not considered as separate individual towns.

Table – No. 8 Growth of Bangalore City during the last 130 years (1871-2001):

Name of the City	Census year	Area	Persons	Male	Females	Sex ratio	Density	0-6 population	Literacy	Decadal variation in per cent
Bangalore UA	1871	NA	144,479	NA	NA	NA	NA	NA	NA	-
	1881	NA	155,857	77,927	87,930	1,128	NA	NA	NA	7.88
	1891	NA	180,366	91,062	89,304	981	NA	NA	NA	15.73
	1901	NA	163,091	83,117	79,974	962	NA	NA	NA	-9.58
	1911	60.35	189,485	97,749	91,736	938	NA	NA	NA	16.18
	1921	NA	240,054	126,784	113,270	893	NA	NA	NA	26.69
	1931	NA	309,785	162,767	147,018	903	NA	NA	52,509	29.05
	1941	NA	410,967	216,340	194,627	900	NA	NA	156,212	32.66
	1951	NA	786,343	417,706	368,637	883	NA	8,979*	335,597	91.34
	1961	501.21	1,206,961	644,047	562,914	874	2,408	NA	597,525	53.49
	1971	177.30	1,664,208	887,782	776,426	875	9,386	NA	908,143	37.88
	1981	365.65	2,921,751	1,541,397	1,380,354	896	7,991	NA	1,856,322	75.56
	1991	445.91	4,130,288	2,170,985	1,959,303	902	9,263	578,560	2820,323	41.36
	2001	531.00@	5,686,844	2,983,926	2,702,918	906	10,710@	624,799	4,340,364	37.69

@ Approximate

* Population in the age group 0-4

Note: The concept of Urban Agglomeration was introduced in 1971. For comparative purposes the aggregated populations of the towns included in UA are given for the various censuses even before 1971.

WARD-WISE POPULATION OF THE BANGALORE CITY CORPORATION, 2001

Bangalore City, Corporation with seven wards was formed in 1949 by merging two independent municipalities' viz., Bangalore City, and Bangalore Cantonment. Since then, the number of wards has been on the increase due to incorporation of surrounding areas on a continuous basis and also due to the ever-increasing population of the city. In the 1971 Census Bangalore City was divided into 63 wards which remained the same in the 1981 Census. In the 1991 Census, Bangalore City had 87 wards and in the 2001 Census the number of wards has gone up to 100.

The Bangalore City Corporation which has 100 wards within its municipal jurisdiction has a population of 4,292,223 accounting for 75.48 per cent of the total population of Bangalore Urban Agglomeration of which 2,240,956 are males and 2,051,267 are females.

The decadal growth rate of population for the decade 1991-2001 for Bangalore City is as high as 61.36 per cent. This high growth rate can be attributed not only to the extension of the municipal limits of Bangalore City but also to the ever increasing population.

The child population in the age-group 0-6 in Bangalore City is 456,325 which constitute 10.63 per cent of the total population of the city as against 13.15 per cent in the 1991 Census.

The sex ratio of the population of the Bangalore City has registered a slight increase from 913 in the 1991 Census to 915 females for every 1000 males in the 2001 Census. However, the sex ratio for the child population of Bangalore City has decreased from 961 in 1991 to 937 in 2001 Census.

In consonance with the overall trend noticed in the State, the literacy rate of Bangalore City's population has increased by 4.20 *per cent*age points in comparison to the 1991 Census. In other words 3,293,853 persons or 85.87

per cent of the population aged 7+ have returned themselves as literates as against 1,886,654 persons or 81.67 *per cent* in the 1991 Census.

Statement 5 gives the ward wise population, child population in age-group 0-6 and literates of Bangalore Municipal Corporation as per 2001 Census.

Ward wise population aged 7+ years, literacy rates and sex ratio will be provided separately.

Padmanabhanagar (Ward No.55) has both the highest male population of 58,842 and the female population of 53,342. Similarly, the lowest male population of 8186 and lowest female population of 7410 are in Moodalapalya (Ward No.38).

In so far as the child population in the age-group 0-6 is concerned, again it is in Padmanabhanagar (Ward No.55) that both the male and female population of 11,800 and 6,011 respectively is highest among other wards of the Bangalore Municipal Corporation. So also, it is low both in case of males (908) and females (905) in Moodalapalya (Ward No.38).

Among the one hundred wards in Bangalore Municipal Corporation area, Chickpet (Ward No.28) and Chandra Layout (Ward No.39) have a extent of 15.90 per cent of its total population in the age-group 0-6. But it is in Sampangiramnagar (Ward No.77) that the content of 0-6 population is as low as 7.41 per cent.

Padmanabhanagar (Ward No.55) has the highest number of both male (46,978) and female (38,136) literates among the other wards of the city. So also Moodalapalya (Ward No.38) has the lowest number of both male (6,518) and female (5,112) literates in Bangalore Municipal Corporation area.

The ward wise literacy rate among the population of Bangalore City varies between a high of 97.78 per cent in Chickpet (Ward No.28) and a low of 66.11 per cent in

Devarajeevanahalli (Ward No.93). Except these two wards all the remaining wards of Bangalore City have a literacy rate of over seventy per cent.

The details regarding the child population in the age-group 0-6 and literates in Bangalore Urban Agglomeration area will be given separately for the year 1971 to 2001.

The concept of urban agglomeration was introduced only in 1971. From then on the population of Bangalore Urban Agglomeration having increased considerably from 1,653,779 in 1971 to 5,686,844 in 2001 an increase of 243.87 per cent over that in 1971, sex ratio being 906 females per I 000 males in 2001.

The population in the age-group 0-6 in Bangalore Urban Agglomeration is 624,799 with 10.99 per cent of its total population. There are 938 female children for every 1000 male children in Bangalore Urban Agglomeration.

The number of literates in Bangalore Urban Agglomeration has increased by more than four fold from 974,067 in 1971 to 4,340,364 an increase of 445.59 per cent over that in 1971. It is interesting to note that the sex ratio among the literates has increased from 679 in 1971 to 821 in 2001. This shows the decadal trend in the increase of female literates.

The population details regarding the major constituent units of Bangalore Urban Agglomeration of 2001 will be given separately.

Apart from Bangalore Municipal Corporation and its outgrowths which contributes 4,303,01 1 persons (75.67 per cent) the significant contribution of population to Bangalore Urban Agglomeration is from the seven City Municipal Councils which is 1,260,284 or 22.16 per cent of the total population of Bangalore Urban Agglomeration.

SLUMS IN KARNATAKA, 2001:

The phenomenon of rapid Urbanisation in conjunction with industrialisation has resulted in the growth of slums. The sprouting of slums occurs due to many factors, such as, the shortage of developed land for housing, the high prices of land beyond the reach of urban poor, a large influx of rural migrants to the cities in search of jobs, etc. In spite of some efforts by the State Governments/UTs to contain the number of slum dwellers, the growth of slums has been increasing rapidly putting tremendous pressure on the existing urban basic services and infrastructure. The existence of slums in urban areas is one of the major problems faced by almost all the metropolitan cities throughout the world and Indian cities are no exception.

The basic characteristics of the slums essentially remain the same i.e. dilapidated and infirm housing structures, poor ventilation, acute over-crowding, and faulty alignment of streets, inadequate lighting, and paucity of safe g water, water-logging during rains, absence of toilet facilities and non-availability of basic physical and social services. The living conditions in slums are usually unhygienic and contrary to all norms of planned urban growth and are an important factor in accelerating transmission of various air and water home diseases.

For the first time, with a view to make available socioeconomic and demographic data for the population living in slums, during the 2001 Census operations, areas considered as slums were formed into separate distinguishable enumeration blocks.

The concept of slums and its definition vary from country to country depending upon the socio-economic conditions of each society. In India, 'Slums' have been defined under Section 3 of the Slums Areas (Improvement and Clearance) Act, 1956. All areas where buildings,

- are in any respect unfit for human habitation;
- are by reason of dilapidation, overcrowding, faulty arrangement and design of such buildings, narrowness or faulty arrangement of streets, lack of ventilation, light,

sanitation facilities or any combination of these factors which are detrimental to safety, health and morals.

In addition to this Central Legislation, every State may have an independent Act where 'Slums' are defined. In Karnataka, the Slum Clearance Board has been constituted for the improvement of slums.

Although it is difficult to define 'Slum', for the purpose o Census of India 2001 it is proposed to treat the following as 'Slum' areas: -

(i) All areas notified as 'Slum' by State/Local Government and UT administration under any Act;

(ii) All areas recognised as 'Slum' by State/Local Government and UT administration which have not been formally notified as slum under any Act;

(iii) A compact area of at least 300 population or about 60-70 households of poorly built congested tenements, in unhygienic environment usually with inadequate infrastructure and lacking in proper sanitary and drinking water facilities. Such areas were identified personally by the concerned Census Charge Officer and also inspected by an officer nominated by the Director of Census Operations.

The slum areas thus have been identified and formed into 2,578 separate blocks in the 2001 Census in 35 statutory towns which had a population of 50,000 or more in the 1991 Census in Karnataka. The names of these towns district wise and the number of 'slum', enumeration blocks with population details are given in statement 8. The numbers of slums as per the 2001 Census in these towns are given in statement 9. It is proposed to tabulate and present Census data for slums separately.

Table – No. 9 Slum Population totals in Karnataka, 2001 (Provisional)

Sl. No	District/ Town	No. of slum enume ration blocks	Population			0-6 population			Literates		
			P	M	F	P	M	F	P	M	F
1	2	3	4	5	6	7	8	9	10	11	12
	Karnataka State	2,578	1,267,759	645,289	622,470	180,157	92,613	87,544	736,229	416,795	319,434
1	Belgaum District	51	26,736	13,498	13.238	4,174	2,129	2,045	13,960	8,216	5,744
	Belgaum (M. Corp.)	23	13,380	6,269	6,111	1,953	997	956	6,505	3,721	2,784
	Nipani (CMC)	3	1,241	604	637	637	91	107	778	441	337
	Gokak (CMC)	25	13,115	6,625	6,490	2,023	1,041	982	6,677	4,054	2,623
2	Bagalkot District	49	22,267	13.639	13,628	4,041	2,155	1,886	13,939	8,213	5,726
	Bagalkot (CMC)	19	10,150	5,074	5,076	1,608	904	704	704	3,202	2,262
	Rabkavi-Banhatti (CMC)	30	17,117	8,565	8,552	2,433	1,251	1,182	1,182	5,011	3,464
3	Buapur District	62	34,548	17,659	16,889	4,890	2,507	2,383	20,857	12,009	8,848
	Buapur (CMC)	62	34,548	17,659	16,889	4,890	2,507	2,383	20,857	12,009	8,848
4	Gulbarga District	55	26,053	13,295	12,758	4,200	2,155	2,045	12,879	7,855	5,024
	Gulbarga (M. Corp.)	55	26,053	13,295	12,758	4,200	2,155	2,045	12,879	7,855	5,024

1	2	3	4	5	6	7	8	9	10	11	12
5	Bidar District	60	34,452	17,766	16,686	5,942	3,092	2,850	21,299	11,980	9,319
	Bidar (CMC)	60	34,452	17,766	16,686	5,942	3,092	2,850	21,299	11,980	9,319
6	Raichur District	126	52,823	26,886	25,937	7,453	3,916	3,537	25,868	15,616	10,252
	Raichur (CMC)	126	52,823	26,886	25,937	7,453	3,916	3,537	25,868	15,616	10,252
7	Koppal District	94	44,695	22,471	22,224	7,148	3,680	3,468	22,130	13,445	8,685
	Gangawati (CMC)	94	44,695	22,471	22,224	7,148	3,680	3,468	22,130	13,445	8,685
8	Gadag District	20	8,644	4,300	4,344	1,372	709	663	4,299	2,508	1,791
	Gangawati (CMC)	20	8,644	4,300	4,344	1,372	709	663	4,299	2,508	1,791
9	Dharwad District	217	107,666	54,725	52,941	15,746	8,203	7,543	61,677	35,346	26,331
	Hubli-Dharwad	217	107,666	54,725	52,941	15,746	8,203	7,543	61,677	35,346	26,331
	(M. Corp.)										
10	Uttara Kannada	12	5,178	2,607	2,571	676	350	326	3,345	1,876	1,469
	District										
	Karwar (CMC)	3	1,598	804	794	219	107	112	983	549	434
	Dandeli (CMC)	9	3,580	1,803	1,777	457	243	214	2,362	1,327	1,035
11	Haveri District	19	9,907	5,022	4,885	1,591	794	797	5,339	3,009	2,330
	Ranibennur (CMC)	19	9,907	5,022	4,885	1,591	794	797	5,339	3,009	2,330

1	2	3	4	5	6	7	8	9	10	11	12
12	Bellary District	314	149,305	76,227	73,078	20,475	10,620	9,055	84,912	50,012	34,900
	Hospet (CMC)	146	67,938	34,738	33,200	8,924	4,653	4,271	39,355	23,078	16,277
	Beellary CMC)	168	81,367	41,489	39,878	11,551	5,967	5,584	45,557	26,934	18,623
13	Chitradurga District	52	27,160	13,734	13,426	3,489	1,772	1,717	18,846	10,169	8,677
	Chitradurga (CMC)	52	27,160	13,734	13,426	3,489	1,772	1,717	18,846	10,169	8,677
14	Davangere District	168	84,696	43,226	41,470	11,948	6,149	5,799	48,656	27,486	21,170
	Davangere (CMC)	148	74,637	38,134	36,503	10,469	5,398	5,071	42,898	24,259	18,639
	Harihar (CMC)	20	10,059	5,092	4,967	1,479	751	728	5,758	3,227	2,531
15	Shimoga District	133	61,292	30,573	30,719	7,947	4,057	3,890	38,162	20,725	17,437
	Shimoga (CMC)	75	32,797	16,336	16,461	4,598	2,373	2,225	19,795	10,549	9,246
	Bhadravathi (CMC)	58	28,495	14,237	14,258	3,349	1,684	1,665	18,367	10,176	8,191
16	Udupi District	-	-	-	-	-	-	-	-	-	-
17	Chikmagalur District	22	9,960	5,024	4,936	1,382	732	650	6,009	3,214	2,795
	Chikmagalur (CMC)	22	9,960	5,024	4,936	1,382	732	650	6,009	3,214	2,795
18	Tumkur District	24	14,035	7,381	6,654	1,774	929	845	9,631	5,375	4,256
	Tumkur (CMC)	24	14,035	7,381	6,654	1,774	929	845	9,631	5,375	4,256
19	Kolar District	88	46,966	23,947	23,019	7,222	3,647	3,575	29,036	16,045	12,991
	RobertsonPet (CMC)	15	7,305	3,597	3,708	930	449	481	5,329	2,820	2,509
	Kolar (CMC)	48	24,977	12,755	12,222	4,113	2,080	2,033	15,794	8,586	7,208

1	2	3	4	5	6	7	8	9	10	11	12
	Chintamani (CMC)	25	14,684	7,595	2,179	2,179	1,118	1,061	7,913	4,639	3,274
20	Bangalore District	733	345,200	177,172	168,028	47,751	24,469	23,282	206,051	115,258	90,793
	Bangalore (M.Corp.)	733	345,200	177,172	168,028	47,751	24,469	23,282	206,051	115,258	90,793
21	Bangalore Rural Dist.	40	22,625	11,572	11,053	3,050	1,596	1,454	12,460	6,990	5,470
	Channapatna (CMC)	9	3,756	1,892	1,864	519	272	247	2,146	1,174	972
	Ramanagaram (CMC)	14	8,281	4,256	4,025	1,231	668	563	4,045	2,180	1,865
	Doddaballapur (CMC)	17	10,588	5,424	5,164	1,300	656	644	6,269	3,636	2,633
22	Mandya District	30	15,759	7,871	7,888	2,085	1,022	1,063	8,527	4,719	3,808
	Mandya (CMC)	30	15,759	7,871	7,888	2,085	1,022	1,063	8,527	4,719	3,808
23	Hassan District	70	38,846	19,605	19,241	4,985	2,548	2,437	26,756	14,254	12,502
	Hassan (CMC)	70	38,846	19,605	19,241	4,985	2,548	2,437	26,756	14,254	12,502
24	Dakshina Kannada District	7	2,394	1,122	1,272	194	113	81	1,933	940	993
	Mangalore (M. Corp.)	7	2,394	1,122	1,272	194	113	81	1,933	940	993
25	Kodagu District	-	-	-	-	-	-	-	-	-	-
26	Mysore District	132	71,552	35,967	35,585	10,622	5,269	5,353	39,658	21,535	18,123
	Mysore (M. Corp.)	132	71,552	35,967	35,585	10,622	5,269	5,353	39,658	21,535	18,123
27	Chamarajanagar Dist.	-	-	-	-	-	-	-	-	-	-

Table – No. 10. Number of Slums in Cities/towns in Karnataka, 2001

Sl. No.	Name of the District	Name of city/town	Total number of Slums as per 2001 Census
1.	Belgaum	Belgaum (M. Corp.) Nipani (CMC) Gokak (CMC)	9 2 13
2.	Bagalkot	Bagalkot (CMC) Rabkavi-Banhatti (CMC)	10 24
3.	Bijapur	Bijapur (CMC)	28
4.	Gulbarga	Gulbarga (M. Corp.)	20
5.	Bidar	Bidar (CMC)	21
6.	Raichur	Raichur (CMC)	42
7.	Koppal	Gangawati (CMC)	27
8.	Gadag	Gadag-Betigeri (CMC)	13
9.	Dharwad	Hubli Dharwad (M. Corp.)	65
10.	Uttara Kannada	Karwar (CMC) Dandeli (CMC)	3 6
11.	Haveri	Ranibennur (CMC)	8
12.	Bellary	Hospet (CMC) Bellary (CMC)	69 47
13.	Chitradurga	Chitradurga (CMC)	16
14.	Davangere	Davangere (CMC) Harihar (CMC)	40 7

15	Shimoga	Shimoga (CMC) Bhadravati (CMC)	29 26
16	Udupi	Nil	0
17	Chikmagalur	Chikmagalur (CMC)	13
18	Tumkur	Tumkur (CMC)	17
19	Kolar	Robertson Pet (CMC) Kolar (CMC) Chintamani (CMC)	5 13 14
20	Bangalore	Bangalore (M. Corp.)	137
21	Bangalore Rural	Channapatna (CMC) Ramanagaram (CMC) Dod Ballapur (CMC)	4 6 5
22	Mandya	Mandya (CMC)	14
23	Hassan	Hassan (CMC)	33
24	Dakshina Kannada	Mangalore (M. Corp.)	6
25	Kodagu	Nil	0
26	Mysore	Mysore (M.Corp.	34
27	Chamraj-nagar	Nil	0
	TOTAL		**826**

Table – No. 11. Number of towns by Civic Status in Karnataka, 2001

District Code	Name of the District	Statutory Towns						Non-Statutory Towns	Total
		Municipal Corporation (M. Crop.)	City Municipal Council (CMC)	Canton-ment Board (CB)	Town Municipal council (TMC)	Town Panchayat (TP)	Notified Area Committe e (NAC)	Census town (CT)	
1	2	3	4	5	6	7	8	9	10
	KARNATAKA	6	40	1	81	90	8	44	270
1	Belgaum	-	2	1	7	6	1	4	22
2	Bagalkot	1	2	-	5	5	-	-	12
3	Bijapur	-	1	-	4	1	-	-	6
4	Gulbarga	1	-	-	6	5	3	2	17
5	Bidar	-	1	-	4	1	-	-	6
6	Raichur	-	1	-	2	3	1	2	9
7	Koppal	-	1	-	1	2	-	1	5
8	Gadag	-	1	-	3	5	-	-	9
9	Dharwad	1	-	-	1	4	-	-	6
10	Uttara Kannada	-	3	-	2	6	-	2	13
11	Haveri	-	1	-	4	3	-	1	9
12	Bellary	-	2	-	1	7	-	1	11
13	Chitradurga	-	1	-	2	3	-	-	6
14	Davangere	-	2	-	-	4	-	-	6

15	Shimoga	-	2	-	2	4	1	-	9
16	Udupi	-	1	-	3	-	-	2	6
17	Chikmagalur	-	1	-	2	5	1	-	9
18	Tumkur		1	-	5	4	-	1	11
19	Kolar		4	-	5	3	-	-	12
20	Bangalore	1	7	-	2	-	-	9	19
21	Bangalore Rural		3	-	5	1	-	1	10
22	Mandya		1	-	3	3	1	-	8
23	Hassan		1	-	4	3	-	1	9
24	Dakshina Kannada	1	-	-	2	5	-	12	20
25	Kodagu		-	-	1	2	-	2	5
26	Mysore	1	-	-	3	4	-	3	11
27	Chamrajnagar			-	2	1	-	-	4

Source: Census Reports, 2001.

Table–No. 12. Statement Showing the Bangalore City Slums details:

Statement Showing the Bangalore City Slums details																	
Sl	Name of the constituency.	Total slums	Percentage	Total Huts	Percentage	Total Population	Percentage	Male	Percentage	Female	Percentage	Sc	Percentage	St	Percentage	Others	Percentage
1	Gandhinagar	17	4.670	2936	2.907	16075	2.672	8264	2.510	7811	2.867	12865	5.478	1186	1.156	2024	0.766
2	Chikpete	8	2.197	1626	1.610	8297	1.379	4184	1.271	4113	1.509	5704	2.429	1165	1.135	1428	0.540
3	Binnipet	19	5.219	8182	8.102	59104	9.826	35530	10.795	23574	8.654	2475	1.054	2930	2.856	53699	20.333
4	Chamaraj pete	30	8.241	7046	6.977	35054	5.828	17860	5.426	17194	6.311	12271	5.225	3454	3.367	19329	7.319
5	Shanthinagar	18	4.945	7853	7.776	29976	4.983	17090	5.192	12886	4.730	6674	2.842	6875	6.703	16427	6.220
6	Basavanagudi	11	3.021	1406	1.392	7084	1.177	3647	1.108	3437	1.261	2707	1.152	1086	1.058	3291	1.246
7	Yalahanka	21	5.769	6143	6.083	37770	6.279	20504	6.229	17266	6.338	12139	5.169	8725	8.507	16906	6.401
8	Jayamahal	21	5.769	4114	4.073	24172	4.018	13117	3.985	11055	4.058	11289	4.807	3294	3.211	9589	3.630
9	Malleswaram	25	6.868	4663	4.617	39745	6.608	19855	6.032	19890	7.301	19794	8.429	12354	12.045	7697	2.914
10	Bharathinagar	24	6.593	3108	3.077	17683	2.939	10140	3.080	7543	2.769	5799	2.469	2682	2.615	9202	3.484
11	Shivajinagar	6	1.648	493	0.488	2976	0.494	1585	0.481	1391	0.510	1793	0.763	384	0.374	799	0.302

12	Jayanagar	46	12.637	12064	11.946	72930	12.125	42465	12.902	30465	11.183	30331	12.916	9075	8.848	33424	12.656
13	Rajaji-nagar	19	5.219	5064	5.014	34096	5.668	17483	5.311	16683	6.124	16707	7.114	2593	2.528	14796	5.602
14	Varthur	33	9.065	8329	8.247	43595	7.248	23912	7.265	19683	7.225	17601	7.495	10452	10.191	15542	5.885
15	Uttara-halli	66	18.131	27959	27.686	172908	28.747	93494	28.406	79414	29.152	76666	32.649	36303	35.397	59939	22.696
	Total	**364**	**100**	**100986**	**100**	**601465**	**100**	**329130**	**100**	**272405**	**100**	**234815**	**100**	**102558**	**10**	**264092**	**100**

The above table brings out the details of slums in Bangalore city as per census 2001, with demographic information such as, area-wise distribution, population, number of huts, caste-wise percentage, etc. There are 364 slums with a population of around 601465 and 100986 huts in about 15 constituencies in the city as a whole. Among all these, Uttarahalli Constituency being the largest constituency in India in terms of area and population covered, has the highest number of slums i.e, 18.13 per cent (66) with 27.68 per cent (27959) of huts with a population of about 28.74 per cent (172908) very closely followed by Jayanagar and Varthur with 12.6 per cent (46) and 9.06 per cent (33) slums, 11.94 per cent (12064) and 8.24 per cent (8329) huts and population of about 12.12 per cent (72930) and 7.24 per cent (43595). Chamarajpet and Malleshwaram follow the above with 8.24 per cent (30) and 6.86 per cent (25) of slums with 6.97 per cent huts and 5.82 per cent population and 4.61 per cent huts and 6.6 per cent of population respectively. This being the higher side of the situation, the other side is Shivajinagar, having only six slums of about 1.6 per cent closely followed by Chickpet having 2.19 per cent (8) of slums with 0.48 per cent of huts and 0.49 per cent of population 1.61 per cent huts and 1.37 per cent population respectively. The other areas are in between these two groups having slums ranging from 24 in Bharathinagar to 11 in Basavanagudi.

Of the total number of huts comparison with total population, Uttarahalli has both highest *per cent* of huts as well as population as already said. The table also brings into picture, the present situation of slums. The basic amenities existing in these slums are far beyond satisfactory and still a lot more has to be done in this direction. The Government has established Slum Clearance Board to take care of the existing and also emerging slums, to provide basic amenities and other required facilities for the residents the benefits are yet to reach maximum number of beneficiaries.

Table – No. 13. Statement Showing the Bangalore City Declared Slums details:

Statement Showing the Bangalore City Declared Slums details													
Sl. No.	Name of the constitu-tency.	No. of slums	Per centage	No. of Huts.	Per centage	No. of Populat ion.	Per centage	SC.	Per cen-tage	ST.	Per centage	Others	Per centage
1	Gandhinagar	12	5.882	1310	3.684	7369	3.214	4749	5.097	1349	3.487	1271	1.306
2	Chikpete	6	2.941	1674	4.708	8611	3.755	4812	5.165	985	2.546	2814	2.891
3	Varthur	21	10.294	4143	11.651	16470	7.183	8320	8.930	2839	7.338	5311	5.456
4	Binnipet	11	5.392	1365	3.839	7620	3.323	2355	2.528	2180	5.635	3085	3.169
5	Jayanagar	23	11.275	1533	4.311	41960	18.299	16606	17.823	3250	8.400	22104	22.707
6	Rajajinagar	7	3.431	1906	5.360	12624	5.505	5708	6.126	3620	9.357	3296	3.386
7	Bharathi-nagar	18	8.824	1533	4.311	9601	4.187	3701	3.972	1803	4.660	4097	4.209
8	Shivajinagar	1	0.490	60	0.169	350	0.153	0	0.000	0	0.000	350	0.360
9	Jayamahal	15	7.353	2009	5.650	12771	5.569	2945	3.161	2060	5.325	7766	7.978
10	Malles-waram	22	10.784	2009	5.650	26467	11.542	11654	12.508	7195	18.597	7618	7.826
11	Badava-nagudi	7	3.431	1464	4.117	7819	3.410	1946	2.089	495	1.279	5378	5.525
12	Yalahanka	12	5.882	3147	8.850	19148	8.350	5595	6.005	3868	9.998	9685	9.949

13	Chamaraj pete	20	9.804	5646	15.877	28040	12.228	9881	10.605	2645	6.837	15514	15.937
14	Shanthinagar	5	2.451	553	1.555	3167	1.381	2094	2.247	110	0.284	963	0.989
15	Uttarahalli	24	11.765	7208	20.270	27288	11.900	12806	13.744	6290	16.258	8092	8.313
	Total	**204**	**100**	**35560**	**100**	**229305**	**100**	**93172**	**100**	**38689**	**100**	**97344**	**100**

The above table tries to unfold the details of declared slums in Bangalore city, with demographic information like, area-wise distribution, population, number of huts, caste-wise percentage, etc. There are 204 declared slums with a population of around 2, 29,305 and 35, 560 huts in about 15 constituencies in the city as a whole. Among all these, Uttarahalli Constituency being the largest constituency in India in terms of area and population covered, has the highest number of slums i.e, 11.76 per cent (24) with 20.27 per cent (7,208) of huts with a population of about 11.9 per cent (27, 288) very closely followed by Jayanagar and Malleshwaram with 11.27 per cent (23) and 10.78 per cent (22) slums. Varthur, Chamarajpet and Bharathinagar follow the above with 10.3 per cent (21), 9.8 per cent (20) and 8.8 per cent (18)of slums with 11.65 per cent huts and 7.18 per cent population, 15.87 per cent huts and 12.22 per cent of population, 4.31 per cent huts and 4.18 per cent population respectively. This being the higher side of the situation, the lower side being Shivajinagar, having only one declared slum of about 0.5 per cent closely followed by Shanthinagar with 2.45 per cent (5) and Chikpete with 2.94 per cent (6) of slums with 0.16 per cent of huts and 0.15 per cent of population, 1.55 per cent huts and 1.38 per centpopulation, 4.7 per cent huts and 3.75 per centpopulation respectively. The other areas coming in between these two categories may be grouped into one ranging from 15 to 7 declared slums Jayamahal at the top with 15 and Basavanagudi and Rajajinagar both at the bottom with 7 slums.

Of the total number of huts when compared with total population, it appears that though Uttarahalli has highest *per cent* of about 20.26 per cent huts, the population is about 11.9 per cent, whereas, Malleshwaram with only 5.64 per cent huts, has almost equal population i.e., of about 11.54 per cent which reflects the high density of population. Similarly Chamarajpet being one of the oldest residential areas in Bangalore has more number of huts and maximum population as said earlier. It is striking to note that Shivajinagar being one of the oldest areas in Bangalore has only one declared slum in spite of having maximum number of slums posing great threat to the development of the area. It can also be noticed that there are no SC/ST population in the Shivajinagar slum as it is Muslim dominated area. A highest, 17.8 per cent of SC population is in Jayanagar slums and a highest, 18.6 per cent of the ST is in Malleshwaram slums. Jayanagar also has the credit of having maximum *per cent* of others of about 22.70 per cent. It can also be noted that the total population of SC and Others in these slums is almost same whereas, the population of ST accounts for only about 40 per cent of their total. The basic amenities existing in these slums are far beyond satisfactory and still a lot more has to be done in this direction. Given this sorry state of declared slums as such, one can imagine the sorry state of affairs in respect of yet to be declared slums. The Government has established Slum Clearance Board to take care of the existing and also emerging slums, to provide basic amenities and other required facilities for the residents the benefits are yet to reach large number of beneficiaries.

Slum Scenario in Bangalore City

Reports on Crime:

a). Vigilance committees to be constituted for slums. The city policy draped their controversial decision to collect details and finger prints of slum dwellers. Instead, they have now decided to help slum dwellers setup 'vigilance committees' to maintain peace in slum. Saying this to reporters here on Friday, city police commissioner H.T.Sangliyana, said, his earlier decision which lead to a debate among the public, in political circle on the press has been completely abandoned. 'It is the duty of slum dwellers to keep criminal away. The vigilance committees will work in that direction we will provide furniture and other facilities to the committees' he said (H.T.Sangliyana) he discussed the issue with slum dwellers who have agreed to it. (*Indian Express*, 5/01/2002).

b). Proposed collection of photos and fingerprints of slum dwellers was dropped amidst severe protest from the slum dwellers and also the public. Based on the information that youngsters from slums are participating in crime activities in the city the proposed act was planned. (*Vijay Karnataka,* 05/01/2002).

c). The writ petition on the collection of photos and finger prints of slum dwellers was cancelled in the High court based on the information that the process has been withheld by the government. (*Samyuktha Karnataka,* 09/01/2002).

d). The Karnataka slum areas (Development and clearance) and related law (Amendment) act 2001. Many people opine that some rules in this act would lead to the misuse of power in the respect of clearance of the areas and many other aspects. (*Prajavani,* 18/01/2002).

Fire Accidents

a). A detailed enquiry about the fire accident in Arundhathi Nagar slum will be done. The people get permanent residence and they will be rehabilitated. The fire accident occurred in the Arundhathi Nagar slum at Gangondanahally on Monday mid night the fire has burnt all the 52 huts in the slum along with all the utensils, cloths and other things of the dwellers. Due to bad road the fire engine could not reach the spot on time. But the enraged public threw stones at the vehicles and damaged them. (*Vijay Karnataka,* 13/03/2002).

b). Bangalore City Development Minister T.John on Thursday gave a compensation of Rs. 5,000 (Five Thousand) each to the sixty families affected in the fire that broke out in Lakshminarayana Slum on Wednesday. Nearly sixty two huts were gutted in the slum at Neelasandra after a couple's tiff turned fiery and the wife, Nandani doused herself with kerosene. The fair subsequently spread to the adjacent huts. While Nandani died, her husband Venkatesh suffered 3rd degree burns while trying to save her. He has been admitted to the Victoria Hospital; his condition is critical. (*Times of India,* 3/05/2002).

Sanitation

The central government has given acceptance for the construction of 1000toilets in the slums of Karnataka under "Nirmala Bharath Abhiyana". Out of 1000,500 will be with in Bangalore slums. Under Vambe and NIrmala Jyothi Projects, 33,000 houses will be constructed for the slum dwellers. (*Vijay Karnataka*, 15/03/2002).

"Kannada News paper for the slum dwellers for 50 paise only"

Paper Movement Organisation has organised a movement in this direction. Out of 1.50 paise cost of Newspaper, 50 paise will be borne by the paper owners, 50 paise by the reader and another 50 paise from the organisation. This was organised to motivate the hobby of reading News paper among the slum dwellers. (*Vijay Karnataka*, 26/03/2002).

Couple's tiff turns fiery: 62 huts gutted:

A couple's marital tiff resulted in 62 huts being gutted in a freak fire accident in Lakshminarayana Rao slum in Adugodi Police Limits (Neelasandra Ward) on Tuesday night. The couple, Venkatesh and Nandini, argued over a domestic issue and in feet of rage, Nandini doused herself with kerosene and set herself ablaze. The fire quickly spread to other huts gutting them. While Nandini died, Venkatesh suffered 3rd Degree burns attempting to save her. He has been admitted to Victoria Hospital and his condition is said to be critical. Fortunately, no other causalities were reported, the police said. The incident left many hut dwellers home less. On Wednesday morning, many were seeing searching the ruble trying to salvage what they could "I have lost everything in the fire and don't know where to go with my children now. Will the government save our life?", asked a victim. It may be recalled that a fire accident was reported in the same slum 15 days ago and about 18 huts were gutted. (*Times of India*, 2/05/2002).

Slum Profiles and Field Observations

1. PANTHARAPALYA:-

This slum is situated in the Bangalore–Mysore highway. It is adjacent to the main road and hence has got many advantages. It is one of the big and noted slums in the city. It has a population of about 3,000. Next to it there is big open drainage running through which pose a great threat to the health and hygiene of the residents. There is also a railway track running through there is an Ashrama to the North of the slum

As for as basic amenities are concerned, the housing condition is very poor, there are no drainage facilities around the houses, toilet facilities are inadequate and unhygienic. Majority of the houses are thatched huts (Kutcha) with only a few houses with asbestos/zinc sheet roofs. There are no proper roads in the slum. All of them are kutcha roads with mud. A big advantage that is available is a Hospital build under India Population Project VIII especially for Women and Children. It provides ante-natal care, post-natal care, immunisation to pregnant women and children, family planning methods like TO/LTO, IUD, OP and CC along with general health care too. The hospital staff also makes field visits to keep track of health conditions of the slum residents. There is a Government primary and higher primary School with classes from 1 to 7 standards. There is free distribution of food grains, books and clothes to the students along with afternoon lunch. In spite there is much difficulty in getting attendance in the classes. Other than this there are two private schools in the slum. The corporation provides tailoring training programme to women from vulnerable sections.

There is no drinking water supply to the slum by the Corporation. It is being supplied by Sri Sathya Sai Baba Trust through Water Tankers. Here, an NGO called 'PARASPARA' is operating a crèche for children below 5 years whose parents go for work. It is also providing awareness to the slum dwellers on health, education, personal hygiene, and capacity building activities for women for organising self help groups. The majority of the people living in this slum are engaged in occupations like manual labour, masonry work, beedi and agarbathi making, etc. There is also a substantiate number of petty vendors. Only 2 per cent of the residents are Government employees. There are 70 per cent of Hindus, 10 per cent Muslims, 5 per cent Christians and remaining 15 per cent others. A Temple and a Church is in the slum.

Field observations

The major problem in this area is open air defecation. There are no public toilet facilities nor do the houses have. The people defecate around the houses and on the either sides of the roads. On the backside of this slum, big open drain passes between the slum and the railway track which carries the drain water collected from all directions. Its width is about 10 ft which causes a stinging smell along with the defecated feces.

The residents say that earlier i.e., about 10 years back, the area was scarcely populated with very few huts. Now the population has increased enormously leading to lack of basic needs. Though the corporation has constructed two public toilets recently, they are hardly used by the public. Women and children never use it whereas; the men rarely make use of it. The reason they give for this is that if a person uses the toilet once he has to pay Rs. 2 which they cannot afford to pay. Hence, though they know that open defecation causes health hazards they have to depend on it without any other go.

2. BAPUJI NAGAR:-

Bapuji Nagar is another slum which is placed adjacent to the Bangalore-Mysore Highway. This is the most developed one among the sample slums. There is a population of about 4,000 in the slum.

Compared to other sample slums, housing conditions and living conditions are higher. Most the houses are RCC roofed (75 per cent-80 per cent). Basic amenities like water supply and drainage are well established. There are public taps, mini water tanks, and also individual taps which cater to the drinking water needs of the people. There are closed drainages around the houses with a big open drainage running along the slum. The garbage is disposed through corporation vehicle which collects it under "Swacha Bengaluru" programme in collaboration with NGOs. There is cleanliness in and around he area but, due to the big open drainage the people are encountered with many health hazards. There are big Temples of Sri Gali Anjaneya Swamy and Sri Beereshwara swamy which attracts a huge number of devotees. The Temple also provides livelihood to the slum residents. They are engaged in activities like flower vending, fruit vending, and other petty shops related to temple activities.

A Government School upto 10th standard and few private schools are operating in the area. A Corporation Hospital is existing which was built under India Population project-VIII and is catering to the health needs of the slum dwellers in general and women and children in particular. It provides ante-natal care, post-natal care, immunisation to pregnant women and children, family planning methods like TO/LTO, IUD, OP and CC along with general health care too. There is a Samudaya Bhavan built by BMP under UBSP Scheme. There are two Anganwadis in the slum. A tailoring class is being run from the Corporation which gives training to the poor women.

'SAMRUDDHI' and 'ASHWA RURAL DEVELOPMENT SOCIETY' are two NGOs operating in this area. Their activities include Capacity Building, Self Help Group formation, Women Empowerment, Health Awareness, etc.

3. RAJIVGANDHI NAGAR:-

This slum is in Peenya Industrial area. By looking at it one gets a picture of rural area/village background. It has a population of around 3,500. Though this slum has existed 10-15 years ago even today it lacks basic amenities like roads, drainages, toilets, drinking water, etc. During rainy season the houses get flooded because of overflowing drainages and create lot of health problems.

Government Hospital is placed at Laggere, which is 2 kms away from the area. For deliveries and other serious problems they have to go to Peenya Dasarahalli. Many private schools are there in the area but with no Government School the slum dwellers are deprived of getting basic education as they cannot afford to send their children to private schools. There are no crèches or Anganwadi for small children to benefit the working class. There are many garment factories around the slum which provides livelihood to them. Most of them are daily wage workers. In these factories women get more employment opportunities.

In this slum ASHWA RURAL DEVELOPMENT SOCIETY has formed SHGs under Nagara Sthree Shakthi Yojane, sponsored by CMC under JSRY scheme, and organizes skill development training programmes. Another NGO is implementing Waste Management Project in assistance with KUIDFC.

Field observations

While returning from the field, a person was fully drunk and all the neighbouring people were gathered near their house. When asked why the reply was, the person who was drunk every day comes and beat his wife and children. The neighbours have tried their level best to mend him with their wordings but in vain. He has replied to them by saying that that they are outsiders and they don't have any rights to advise him. According to the neighbours, that person does not do any work and he snatches away the wife's earnings every day, drink and beat wife and children mercilessly. They have four children. Of them, two go to the nearby Government School and the other two go for work. Their earnings are not sufficient for their father's drinking. There are no proper clothes to wear and even food to eat. When asked to him about why he does like this, he said that he is a menial labour who cleans the blocked sewage pipes. To keep himself unaware of the nasty smell while working he is addicted to drinking. His hut is small, thatched with a living space of 10X10. There are six members in the family, husband, wife and four children. When I visited them he had beaten his wife and she was crying sitting in a corner surrounded by two small children of whom one was hit by him while beating wife as he came in between.

In the afternoon during lunch time, a pregnant lady came to the Government hospital where I was waiting to have discussions with the Lady Medical Officer. Since the Doctor had gone to the Anganwadi to put immunisation to the children, she had to wait till her arrival. In the mean time I had a chance to discuss with that lady. She is a housewife, has three female children and due to want of male child by her husband and in-laws she is pregnant again. There is no proper spacing between the children due to lack of awareness and also blind belief that use of such methods may lead to inability to beget child or may lead to disorders in the child. All the three children are partially immunised. The lady was under nourished; though her age was about 25-26 she appeared like 35-40 years old due to over burden she had from continuous deliveries and responsibility of taking care of three children at a time.

In this area the roads are broader in width but in vain as they are not tarred, full of mud and stones which hiders the smooth movement of vehicles including people. The houses are scarcely built and there is lot of vacant space around the houses. This has created small bushy places facilitating the breeding of pigs, bandicoots, dogs and even snakes. These animals roam fearlessly on the roads and pose great threat to the children and women apart from causing health problems. One has to travel a minimum of about 3-4 kms to get treatment as there is no Government Hospital nearby. The corporation has not made any efforts to control the menace of these animals.

4. ATHMAJYOTHI NAGAR:-

This slum exists behind Pantharapalya slum. The living conditions are worse than that of the Pantharapalya. The population of the slum is about 2500. Except Schools, other basic amenities likc, drinking water, drainages and roads are better placed in comparison with Pantharapalya. Housing conditions too are better as this is relatively new and hence most of the houses are pucca houses with sheets. The Corporation has to pay attention towards this slum and should try to make it in to a developed one at the earliest. This could be easier at this stage as the area is still under development.

'PRARASPARA' trust, an NGO in Pantharapalya is trying to extend its area of operation to this slum too and is in the initial stages of working.

5. CHOWDESHWARI NAGAR:-

This slum is situated in Peenya Dasarahalli industrial area. It is 12 kms away from the Bangalore city adjacent to outer ring road. This is one of the most backward slums among the sample. Except drinking water being provided under 11th Five year Plan all other basic amenities are yet to be addressed. The houses are pucca houses with Sheets and also RCC roofing as most of the houses are owned by middle class people. There are no proper roads in the area. Only 5 per centof the roads are tarred it is even difficult for the two wheelers to travel during rainy season as the existing mud roads skid and vehicles could hardly move on them.

The Government hospital does not exist. One should go to Laggere for getting treatment in Government hospital. Two or three private clinics are there to cater at emergency. There are no Government schools. Private schools are there to which the parents has to send their children if they wish to educate them.

Field observations

Chowdeshwari Nagar is adjacent to Laggere. There are no modern amenities in this area. The corporation water comes once in two days that too in the afternoon when most of the residents are away for earning their livelihoods. If they stay back to collect the water they lose their bread and vice-versa. They struggle for water like anything.

Roads are another menace which troubles the residents a lot. There are no tarred-roads in this area. All are kutcha roads with mud and stones, full of pits and humps. During rainy season even cycling becomes dangerous, not to speak of two-wheelers.

There are no drainages and even if exist, of no use as they have virtually been closed. The drain water stagnates in the pits and holes existing in the roads near the house and becomes breeding place for mosquitoes and other flies causing serious health hazards.

The existing transport facilities are insufficient and inadequate to meet the needs of the public. One has to walk at least one kilometer to catch the bus. There are no proper timings for the bus. It depends on the driver and conductor's will and wishes.

Water comes once in two days very irregularly. Open drainages are not cleaned they are silted and blocked. Roads are in the same condition as they were 12 years ago even today.

When heavy rains occur, the whole Rajiv Gandhi Nagar fills with water. Even the houses drown in water. It takes 3-4 days to come out of the situation.

Bus facilities are very poor. One has to wait hours together to get buses. There are no proper timings for the buses and frequency too is very less.

Water that comes is of very poor quality. Greenish coloured water is supplied which poses a great threat to the health conditions of the people. The tank near by is filled with silt and if it is desilted and cleaned, the water problem of the area may be solved.

There is no Corporation School and Hospital nearby. One has to go 3-4 kms for this. It is very difficult and dangerous too to walk about in the evenings as there is no street lights available and even if present, they are very scanty in number and are placed very spaciously which hardly could provide any lighting during the nights. Due to this the criminal activities are more in nights and hence, women folk can't move out after the day time. Added to this, the problems like street dogs, bandicoots, and pigs etc make the surrounding environment more hazardous. The Corporation seems to have forgotten to spray the medicines in the area.

Near Water Tank: The water tank is multi purpose in the sense that though it is exclusively meant for supply of drinking water, the same is also being used for other domestic purposes like cleaning utensils and washing clothes. There is no proper drainage for passage of water that falls on the ground around the tank. The water stagnates in a pothole next to the tank and serves as breeding place for mosquitoes and flies. The residents disclosed that there is no other place for washing clothes and if they wish to wash near their house, the water would stop before they store according to their necessity. By doing all the work near the tank, they can complete before the water gets over. Another problem is that they should complete their work in time to go for the work and if they don't do it they get delayed for the work and also there is a possibility of pending of the domestic works which causes problem to them after coming home from the work. If the water comes during their working hours they cannot store water even for drinking purpose. The tank water is even used for bathing purpose including brushing and washing face.

When enquired about the health hazards caused by the stagnant water near the tank, they replied that so far they have not come across any such problems and they suffer from common problems like cough, cold and fever with rare cases of viral infection, diarrhea, etc.

The elected representatives never turn back till next elections and the people hardly get any chance to convey their problems to any person.

Socio-economic Background of Sample Slum Population:

Commenting on the growth of urban sociology, Dhavagere observes, "studies of slums conducted by A.R. Desai and Devadas pillai (1972), and by victor D'Souza (1970-74) constitute a separate category within the area of city studies but good studies on the social background of slum-dwellers, pattern of their settlement, slum organisation and so on are very few" (1993, 60).

a) Social background of the sample of the slum population constitutes an important and integral part of the present theses. Concerned with the environmental charges that have accompanied the proliferation of slums an attempt has been made to analyze the variables that constitute the social background of the sample of respondents. Sociological thinking holds the view that mode of existence – 'the social being' determines the social consciousness which in turn determine the manner in which people perceive and actually respond to environmental changes. "Human causes of environmental changes and human reaction to these changes" (Egberttellegen And Martin Wolsink, 1994, Pp.2) is the core of subject matter of environmental sociology in particular and other Behavioural sciences in general. A careful consideration of variable that constitute social background of the sample cannot be over-emphasised. Most environmental changes whether positive of negative are essentially anthropogenetic changes. Study of dynamics of human behaviour occupies a pre-eminent place in the analysis of impact assessment of environmental changes.

b) Each of these variables and the manner in which they interact with one another has been examined across all the five slums. This would help to gain certain insights into the actual behaviour of slum people which would impinge on the environment and consequently certain environmental changes occur. Experience has shown that most environmental changes that have hither to occur have been largely negative. Knowingly and unknowingly human beings have been responsible for this. There can not be a healthy population in an unhealthy environment. Slums represent extreme forms of social disorganisation and environmental and ecological ramifications of social disorganisation have got to be carefully studied. An analysis of social background of sample of slum dwellers becomes absolutely essential in a study like the present one. Social world is generally understood in terms of relations of variables.

c) Peter Blau, the chief exponent of macro-structuralism, argues that variables can interplay with one another in different ways under different circumstances. He argues in terms of what he calls, 'consolidation of parameters' and 'intersection of parameters'. The former happens in social structures in which human beings depend upon one another in the least possible ways and hence the degree and frequency of interactions are extremely limited and hence social relations tend to become rigid and hierarchical and social mobility is extremely limited and greater socio-economic disparities persist. Whereas, the latter happens when human beings depend upon one another to a far greater extent and tend to enter into diverse social-relations and there will be greater frequency of interaction and social relations tend to become flexible and open-ended and socio-economic disparities if any are limited to differences in their respective social functions. By means of different combinations and permutations of social variables, Peter Blau attempts to explain the dynamics of social behaviour. An analysis of social variables and interaction that occurs across variables enables us to understand better the determinants of social behaviour.

The variables included in the study are, a) Occupational composition, b) Educational composition, c) Income, d) Age composition, e) Sex composition, f) Caste composition, g) Religious composition, h) Family sizc, i) Place of residence, j) Housing conditions, k) Migration profile, etc.

a) The concepts of occupation has bee most extensively used in sociology. Given the extremely limited range of variation of occupations we can do no better than adopting Max Weber's classification of manual occupation into–skilled manual workers; Semi-skilled Manual workers; unskilled manual workers and the poor-because of grossly disadvantageous life chances, due to weak or marginal position in the labour market.

Slum people have been known for engaging themselves almost out of necessity in certain economic activities which are predominantly menial, manual, unskilled, and semi-skilled. These activities however useful for them to earn the livelihood will produce certain consequence which if unchecked would adversely affect environment. For example: Tanning activities have exposed people working there in to grave health risks like wide variety of allergic skin complications. Beedi workers' children contract bronchi disease due to their constant exposure to tobacco, to mention a few. Given these possibilities the data analysis regarding occupational composition of the sample acquires a special importance. Unskilled Manual Wage Labourers (construction, domestic worker, toilet cleaning, drainage cleaning, road cleaning, loading and unloading, agriculture and gardening, etc.), Skilled Manual Labourers (painter, mason, electrician, mechanic, carpenter, leather worker, beedi, agarabathi making, plumber, doll making and zary work etc.), semi-skilled manual worker–government workers, Service workers and petty business (vegetable vendor, ice candy vendor, balloon vendor and paper vendors, etc.), Business (Tailoring shop, Ration shop, Electric shop, Chicken and mutton centre, STD Shop, etc.,), Teacher, Sales men, house wife, government employees and host of other lower level and subordinate services.

It can be seen from the table-1 that majority of the sample in all the five slums is engaged in manual work and occupation, while far less proportion of the sample reported to have engaged in service occupations like teaching, sales, working at home and government employment to mention a few. Theories of Urbanisation argue that increase in Urbanisation is accompanied by a shift in the occupational distribution of population. The shift takes place from agriculture and allied manual primary occupations to predominantly service occupation like education research, health, transport, communication, hotel and entertainment to mention but a few examples. It is indeed surprising to note that slum population in Bangalore city continues to depend upon and actually find employment only in primary activities.

This finding is hardly surprising and reflects the social character of Urbanisation in India. Bulk of slum dwellers are migrants having been pushed out of their villages due to severe drought conditions prevailing in rural Karnataka particularly the neighbouring districts of Bangalore city. This further reinforces the impression that increase in urban population is due to increase of the slum population due to unabated proliferation of slums. So much so, the disparities in urban population have become increasingly visible with serious implications for social integrity in towns and cities. On the one hand a vast mass of disempowered, property less sick unhygienic poor and on the other extremely rich affluent classes. Given the phenomenal increase in the size of urban poor and the inability of the Government and municipal administration to meet their basic needs the unprecedented pressure on urban infrastructure is inevitable and the environmental degradation that follows has disastrous consequences.

Analysis of data brings out the nature of interaction between Urbanisation, increase in the size of slum population in particular and urban poor in general and the environmental degradation. There has been steady decline in the quality of life of urban residents. On the one hand urban poor tend to suffer from the scarcities of basic needs and hence, have become increasingly vulnerable to various health hazards and on the other the increase in the affluence of minorities of urban rich with fast changing lifestyles have also become extremely vulnerable to stress-related psycho-somatic health disorders. Environmental degradation has further aggravated these problems. What is the way out of this predicament is a matter of serious concern.

Table No. 14 - Occupational composition

Sl.No	Name of the slum.	Manual Wage Laborer	Skilled Laborer	Petty Business	Business.	Factory Worker.	Teacher	Sales	At home/house wife	Student	Government employee	Unemployed	Total
1	B.Nagar	7	16	5	10	8	0	1	2	0	1	0	50
2	R.J Nagar	6	25	5	4	8	0	0	1	0	1	0	50
3	P. Palya	23	18	5	0	2	0	0	0	0	2	0	50
4	A.J. Nagar	31	10	2	1	2	0	1	1	0	1	1	50
5	C. Nagar	1	26	2	5	3	1	5	2	0	4	1	50
6	All slums	68	95	19	20	23	1	7	6	0	9	2	250

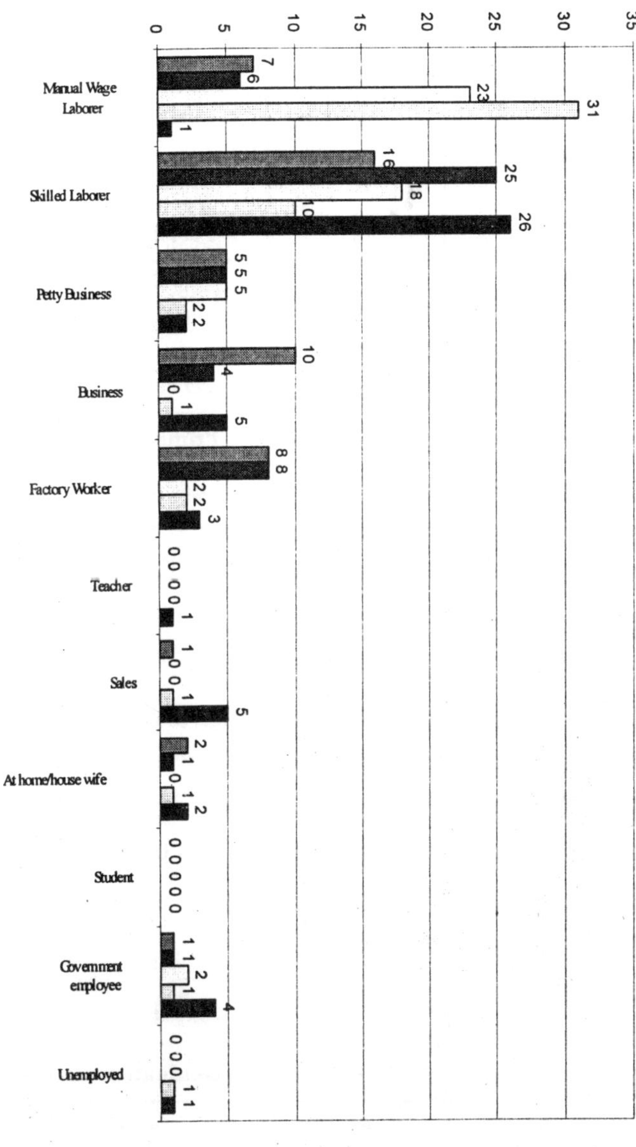
Manual Wage Laborer
Skilled Laborer
Petty Business
Business
Factory Worker
Teacher
Sales
At home/house wife
Student
Government employee
Unemployed
0
5
10
15
20
25
30
35
1 B. Nagar
2 R.J Nagar
3 P. Palya
4 A.J. Nagar
5 C. Nagar

Table No. 15 - Educational Composition:

Sl. No	Name of the slums	Illiterates	*Per centage*	Literates informal education	*Per centage*	Primary 1-4	*Per centage*	Middle school 5-7	*Per centage*	High school 8-10	*Per centage*	PUC	*Per centage*	Diploma	*Per centage*	Graduation	*Per centage*	Post graduation	*Per centage*
1	B. Nagar	10	20	8	16	8	16	4	8	12	24	6	12	1	2	0	0	1	2
2	R. Nagar	9	18	0	0	3	6	5	10	26	52	5	10	0	0	2	4	0	0
3	P. Palya	25	50	0	0	5	10	9	18	10	20	1	2	0	0	0	0	0	0
4	A.J. Nagar	32	64	0	0	3	6	2	4	11	22	0	0	0	0	2	4	0	0
5	C.Nagar	7	14	1	2	2	4	9	18	25	50	2	4	0	0	3	6	1	2
All slums		83	33	9	4	21	8	29	12	84	34	14	6	1	0	7	3	2	0.8

Having discussed occupational composition, we will now turn to discuss educational composition. It is widely believed that slum people are illiterates, uneducated and show less inclination towards opportunities to get education. This picture has prevailed, no doubt, for a very long time. It is indeed surprising to note that educational level of lower class and lower caste people has been gradually rising.

It can be seen in the table-2 that 34 per cent of sample are educated up to high school and 33.2 per cent of sample are illiterates though we notice some significant variation across the five slums. 7 per cent of the sample has studied up to graduation and there is nobody in professional education. This data has certain implications like, even though 34 per cent of sample have studied up to high school almost the same *per cent*age still remain illiterates this means that literacy spreads very slowly and that very few people have been able to get into college education and the so called professional education remains outside the reach of slum population. Almost all theories of development consistently argue that education is the single most important factor for socio-economic development of people who belong to weaker sections of society. Even though government claims to have extended the benefits of education to slum people in particular and urban poor in general, it appears to have made only a marginal impact. Illiterates are those who do not know how to read and write and hence are the most gullible lot of the slum. Non government organisations also often claim to concentrate their efforts in giving education to poor people but, the data do not bare it out. Not withstanding their sufficient exposure to urban life the mission of education is yet to reach the slums. Slum people continue to live on the border lines of dirt, disease, and disabilities. There are still enough of opportunities for people who want to take education to slums. Baring primary education the so called government funded higher education is yet to reach the urban poor.

While privatisation and commercialisation of professional and technical education is increasing and becoming almost

Table No. 16 Age composition

Sl. No	Name of the slum	15-20	Per centage	21-25	Per centage	26-30	Per centage	31-35	Per centage	36-40	Per centage	41-45	Per centage	46-50	Per centage	50 and above	Per centage
1	B.Nagar	0	0	1	2	11	22	9	18	7	14	9	18	5	10	8	16
2	R.J.Nagar	0	0	3	6	19	38	11	22	6	12	6	12	3	6	2	4
3	P.Palya	0	0	6	12	13	26	15	30	5	10	5	10	3	6	3	6
4	A.J.Nagar	1	2	5	10	8	16	11	22	9	18	10	20	1	2	5	10
5	C.Nagar	0	0	5	10	12	24	9	18	12	24	5	10	3	6	4	8
	All slums	1	0.4	20	8	63	25.2	55	22	39	15.6	35	14	15	6	22	8.8

the monopoly of well to do sections of the society, it is only the rich and upper classes who can offer costly medical and management education. Primarily, education which is highly elitist is controlled by the big business houses. Education instead of serving as a means of reducing socio-economic disparities has turned to be a means of ever widening socio-economic disparities. Not withstanding the universalisation of education promised in the Indian Constitution, education in contemporary India has become the most contentious issue.

In our tradition, generally the elderly person assumes the position of Head of the family. In the changed scenario from joint to nuclear families today, we can see maximum *per cent* assuming the role of Head of the family in the age group of 21to 40 amounting to more than 70 per cent. The table projects the fact that the maximum number of head of the families are in the age group 26-30 of about 25.2 per cent followed by 31-35 around 22 per cent and 36-40 summing to 15.6 per cent. There is only one person in the age group of 15-20 i.e., 0.4 per cent. The remaining sample comes under the age group 21-25 of 8 per cent, 41-45 of 14 per cent and above 50 of 8.8 per cent.

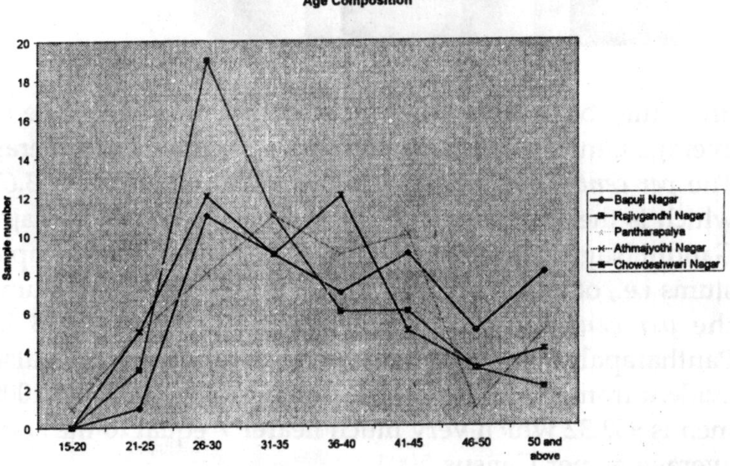

Table No. 17 - Sex Composition / Family Size					
Sl.No	Name of the slum	Location	Male	Female	Total
1	B. Nagar	Binnipet	122	107	229
2	R.J. Nagar	Peenya	94	87	181
3	P. Palya	Mysore road	104	85	189
4	A.J. Nagar	Uttara halli	118	123	241
5	C. Nagar	Hegganahalli	96	98	194
All slums		Bangalore	534	500	1034

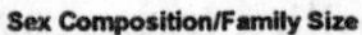

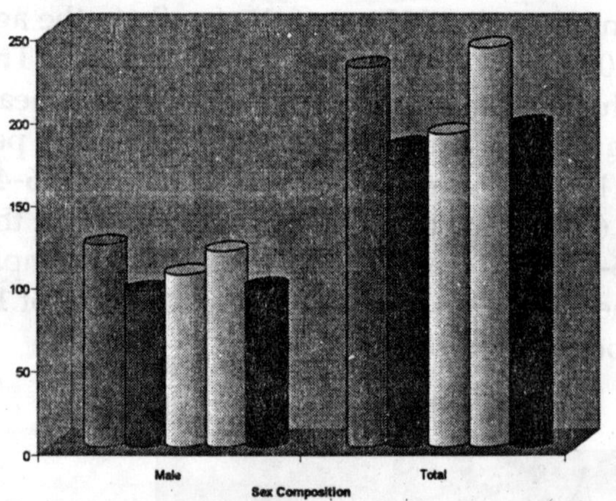

From the above table it can be seen that the *per cent*age of average family size is around four (4) members in general. The *per cent*age of average family size ranges from 3.62 which is the lowest among the sample slums i.e., of Rajiv Gandhi Nagar and 4.82 which is highest among the sample slums i.e., of Athma Jyothi Nagar. In the remaining slums the *per cent* range is 4.58 in Bapuji Nagar, 3.78 in Pantharapalya, and 3.88 in Chowdeshwari Nagar. It is also evident from the table that the number of women per 1000 men is 932.32 which very much nearer / equal to the state average as per Census 2001.

Table No. 18 - Household Income:

Sl.No	Name of the slum	Less than 1000	1001 to 2500	2501 to 5000	5001 to 7500	7501 to 10000	Above 10000	Nil	Total
1	B. Nagar	3	20	17	4	6	0	0	50
2	R. Nagar	2	10	32	5	0	0	1	50
3	P. Palya	3	34	13	0	0	0	0	50
4	A. Nagar	1	19	22	6	2	0	0	50
5	C. Nagar	0	11	29	8	2	0	0	50
6	All slums	9	94	113	23	10	0	1	250

Keeping in view, the skill component of the slum people and the nature of occupation in which slum people engage themselves and the demand for such labour in the labour market, we have arrived at the following classification of income groups. It does not tally with the income groups among non-slum urban population.

Table No. 19 - Income groups

Sl.No	Income groups	Amount (Rs)	Total	*Per centage*
1	Least income	Less than 1000	9	3.6
2	Low income	1001to 2500	94	37.6
3	Lower-middle income	2501 to 5000	113	45.2
4	Middle-middle income	5001 to 7500	23	9.2
5	Upper-middle income	7501 to 10000	10	4
6	Upper income	Above 10000	0	0
7	No income	0	1	0.4
		Grand total	**250**	**100**

Household Income is another variable considered to describe social background. In case of unorganised sector, assessing income is one of the difficult and ticklish issues. It is because not only people in the unorganised sector will have no regular income, but also they have no way of keeping track of their income. Yet this variable cannot be ignored. Income gives us some idea regarding economic status of population. For clarity we have divided the sample into the following income groups:

1. Lowest income group, members who earn less than Rs.1,000 per month
2. Low income group, members who earn between Rs.1,001 and 2,500 per month
3. Lower-middle income group, members who earn between Rs.2,501 and 5,000 per month
4. Middle income group, members who earn between Rs.5,001 and 7,500 per month
5. Upper-middle income group, members who earn between Rs.7,501 and 10,000 per month

It can be noted from the table that no one reported to earn above Rs.10,000. Expectedly middle income group constitute 45.2 per cent of the total sample followed by 37.6 per cent of the sample belonging to low income group. It appears from the table that least *per cent*age of the sample 3.6 per cent belong to the least income. The data shows that there has been some increase in the income of slum people given the building construction boom. A large number of people from low income group not only find work regularly but also they are able to earn if not adequate income but income which is barley sufficient to meet their basic needs. Given the increasing the cost of living and the rise in prices of the essential goods and services, the income 2,501 and 5,000 is not sufficient. Only 4 per cent of the sample reported to have monthly income up to 10,000.

Table No. 20 - Caste *per centage*

Sl.No	Name of the slum	Name of the Caste and Per centage															
		Vyshyas	per cent	Balajiga	per cent	Lingayath	per cent	Brahmins	per cent	Gowdas/ Vakkaliga	per cent	Muslims	per cent	Mudaliyars	per cent	Maraties	per cent	S/c	per cent
1	B. Nagar	0	0	1	2	0	0	0	0	5	10	1	2	0	0	0	0	35	70
2	R.J. Nagar	3	6	6	12	0	0	0	0	19	38	0	0	5	10	1	2	4	8
3	P. Palya	1	2	3	6	0	0	0	0	3	6	1	2	0	0	0	0	37	74
4	A.J. Nagar	0	0	1	2	0	0	0	0	5	10	1	2	0	0	0	0	35	70
5	C. Nagar	2	4	3	6	0	0	1	2	18	36	2	4	2	4	0	0	10	20
All slums		**6**	**2.4**	**14**	**5.6**	**0**	**0**	**1**	**0.4**	**50**	**20**	**5**	**2**	**7**	**2.8**	**1**	**0.4**	**121**	**48.4**

Ganigashetty	0	3	0	0	0	3
per cent	0	6	0	0	0	1.2
St	5	2	1	5	1	14
per cent	10	4	2	10	2	5.6
Srivaishna vas	0	1	0	0	0	1
per cent	0	2	0	0	0	0.4
Madival	0	1	0	0	0	1
per cent	0	2	0	0	0	0.4
Thogata veera	0	1	0	0	0	1
per cent	0	2	0	0	0	0.4
Achars	0	2	0	0	1	3
per cent	0	4	0	0	2	1.2
Setu(Jain)	0	1	0	0	1	2
per cent	0	2	0	0	2	0.8
Kuruba	0	0	0	0	1	1
per cent	0	0	0	0	2	0.4
Christian	3	0	3	3	2	11
per cent	6	0	6	6	4	22
Edigas	0	1	0	0	2	3
per cent	0	2	0	0	4	1.2
Golla	0	0	1	0	0	1
per cent	0	0	2	0	0	0.4
Kumbara	0	0	0	0	1	1
per cent	0	0	0	0	2	0.4
Kshathriyas	0	0	0	0	2	4
per cent	0	0	0	0	4	1.6
Bajanthri	0	0	0	0	1	1
per cent	0	0	0	0	2	0.4

Table No. 21 - Caste composition				
Sl. No	**Status of castes**	**Castes**	**Tota l**	**Per centage**
1	Upper castes	Brahmins , Lingayaths and Vyshyas,	2	0.8
2	Upper Middle castes	Vakkaliga,	8	3.2
3	Middle	Balajigas, Mudaliyars, Edigas, Kurabas, Achars and Maraties.	66	26.4
4	Lower middle castes	Ganigas, Thogataveeras, Gollas, Mdivalas, Muslims Christians, Kumbara, Bajanthri,	39	15.6
5	Low castes	Scheduled castes and Scheduled tribes	135	54
		Grand total	250	100

Caste composition is another important and interesting aspect of the sample population. Theoretically and empirically institution of caste has been the most extensively researched aspect of the Indian society. M. N. Srinivas, the Doyen of Indian sociology, remarked, "caste dies hard in Indian society." Nearly more than half-a-century of modernisation has not disproved it. Historically caste system has defied those who want to understand it and defeated those who want to remove it. No sociological study is complete without a detailed discussion of the institution of caste. Theories of caste system hold the view that it is essentially hierarchical in character and based on the notion 'purity and pollution'. Accordingly, caste groups are differentially located in social space. So much so that the top order is occupied by the so called Sanskritsed caste while middle order is occupied by wide range of intermediary castes. The lower order is occupied by low castes which are traditionally neglected, disempowered and dispossessed. Studies have been made to see whether changes have taken place at the base and if so the direction in which such changes is taking place and the implications thereof for the Indian society. Be it as it may, an attempt is made here to examine the distribution of caste across the five slums. For purpose of analysis various castes in the sample have been divided into a) Upper castes, which include Brahmins, Lingayaths and Vysyas. b) Upper middle castes which includes Vakkaliga, c) Middle castes which include Balajigas, Mudaliyars, Edigas, Kurabas, Achars and Maraties. d) Lower middle castes which include, Ganigas, Thogataveeras, Golla, Madivala and Christian and e) Low caste which includes Scheduled Castes and Scheduled Tribes. One thing that strikes immediately is that almost all castes which are found in wider and main stream society have been reflected obviously though in different *per cent*age across the five slums. Yet it could be noted that Brahmins are found in the least number i.e., only a single household each in Atmajyothi Nagar and Chowdeshwari Nagar and they are not found in the other three slums. One could hazard a guess whether this has something to do with development status of the slums. The data drawn from the sample does not seem to bear this out that upper caste people are not necessarily attracted to developed slums because a person may be caste-wise superior but economically and politically weak. In the present sample, Bapuji Nagar slum is a developed slum because, it is located very close to Bangalore - Mysore highway road. It has tar roads, drainages, good schools, hospitals, transport and communication facilities, and people in that slum have access to all civic amenities and also corporation collects garbage and solid waste. So much so, for all practical purposes it has got assimilated into and integrated with the main city even though officially it is a declared slum. It may be argued, however, that availability of civic amenities alone can not be regarded as indices of development and that alone cannot ensure improvement in quality of life of the people. Development also depends upon how people actually make use of these facilities to be able to achieve improvement in the quality of life. Argued in this way, cultural changes constitute a prelude to over all development. Cultural changes seem to be far too marginal and slum people have got to go a long way in this direction.

The data also shows that low caste people alone need not necessarily live in slums as it has hitherto been believed. It means that over a period of time there have been some changes in the social composition of slum population. This also shows that people struggle hard to have a place to live and for having roof over their head. Atmajyothi Nagar slum is regarded as less developed because, there not only civic amenities are inadequate but, also the existing facilities are in bad shape. Pantharapalya, Chowdeshwari Nagar and Rajiv Gandhi Nagar Slums are underdeveloped because, the civic amenities made available in the other two slums are conspicuous by their absence. Irrespective of level of development people belonging to all castes are found in the sample. It is no longer true to believe that only low caste and backward castes alone live in slums.

References

1. *Census Reports*, 2001.
2. 1 Dhadave, M.S. 1988, *Sociology of Slum*, Archives Books, New Delhi-55.
3. Egberttellegen and Martin Wolsink, University of Amsterdam, Netherlands.
4. 1994: *Society - Its Environment*, Gordon and Breach Science Publishers.
5. *Vijay Karnataka*, 05/01/2002.
6. *Samyuktha Karnataka*, 09/01/2002.
7. *Prajavani*, 18/01/2002.
8. *Vijay Karnataka*, 13/03/2002.
9. *Vijay Karnataka*, 15/03/2002.
10. *Vijay Karnataka*, 26/03/2000.
11. *Times of India*, 2/05/2002.
12. *Times of India*, 3/05/2002.

CHAPTER IV

SLUM AND LIVING ENVIRONMENT OF SLUM DWELLERS AND ITS IMPACT ON URBAN LIFE

The most pressing environmental health problems today, in terms of disease, illness, disabilities and even death are associated with poor households and communities in the developing world. In rural areas and in the peri-urban slums of the developing world, inadequate shelter, overcrowding, lack of adequate safe drinking water and sanitation, contaminated food, and indoor pollution are by far the greatest environmental threats to human health. These conditions are often compounded by poor nutrition and lack of education, which make people more vulnerable to, and less able to cope with, environmental threats.

According to WHO and the World Bank, environmental improvements at the household and community level would make the greatest difference for global health. Specifically, the World Bank has calculated that improvements in local environmental conditions facing the poor could lower the incidence of major killer diseases by up to 40 per cent.

Given the strong correlation between environmental health risks and poverty, one strategy to reduce these risks is to raise incomes and improve the distribution of opportunities, political power and economic resources. Without question, reducing poverty and closing the gap between rich and poor would drastically lower the toll of death and disability from many diseases. Implementing policies to eradicate poverty remains a top priority for improving health, and many organisations-including national governments, the United Nations (U.N.), numerous non-governmental organisations (NGOs), and foundations - have marshaled considerable force toward this end. (The United Nations Development Programme (UNDP) *Human Development Report, 1997)*

Action based strategies aim at empowering the poor in general and local people in managing the resources and distribution of benefits of economic growth. Another argument that has often been put forth by development sociologists revolve around the interface between environmental management and economic development. That development can't be compromised for the sake of protecting the environment just for the sake of doing so. Experience has shown that economic development irrespective the system in which it is sought to be promoted resulted in environmental destruction even though the destruction is most visible under the capitalist style of development. Environmentally sensitive and socially sensible development theorists have pleaded for promoting what has come to be known 'sustainable development' – a development model. As a process it seeks to maintain balance between environmental management and socio-economic development in which the development needs of not only the present but future generation are taken into consideration and maintaining social equality. Environmental management and economic development must go hand in hand reaches a certain level, however; it is a critical tool for improving public health not only present but also future. By implementing policies that help reduce environmental threats it is possible to improve quality of life long before income growth could do so on its own. Improving the conditions of daily life may by itself help to reduce poverty. Removing the environmental hazards that make people sick could keep people working and raise incomes.

Many of the interventions particularly in the domain public health rely on changes in behaviour and improvements in the environment at the household level, because a large share of disease is incurred in or around the home environment. For instance, even if water supplies are clean at the public tap, they can become contaminated if stored in an unhygienic manner. This reality makes the role of public policy difficult, since policies are generally directed toward the public domain. One key role for public action is investment in health and hygiene education. Several studies have shown that the promotion of hand washing, for instance, can drastically reduce the incidence of diarrheal diseases. In addition, abundant evidence has made it clear that educating women more broadly has an immediate positive effect on health.

Policy actions should not be limited to education alone. Governments and non-governmental organisations can also help facilitate changes at the household level by removing many of the institutional and financial barriers that keep poor households from protecting themselves. As one scholar has explained, "The poor lack healthy water systems only because they cannot afford them, but also because they lack the political space to organize and the political leverage to make the public sector respond to their needs." To remove such barriers, governments can develop financing schemes that offset the initial investments needed to improve coverage of basic infrastructure for low-income communities. In addition, both governmental and development agencies should ensure that primary health care packages include environmental interventions as a key component. In other words, health care packages should provide access to water filters, polystyrene beads, and bed nets - all useful to prevent exposure to infectious agents as well as to vaccines and drugs.

The low quality of life in slums is as much a result of unhygienic living conditions as it is of the lack of economic resources. Squalor accompanied by outbreak of diseases, high mortality and general ill health makes slum dwellers become much less productive. To improve the slum environment, Ankur a voluntary organisation along with other agencies probed the socio-economic reasons, which breed an environment un-conducive to healthy living, as also the ways to remedy it.

Living environment of slum dwellers:

Living environment means the actual concrete living conditions which among other things, includes the material used to construct houses, the type of houses, the living space, house hold hygiene, personal hygiene, sexual life, use and storage of water and a host or other material conditions of existence not to speak of the type of food slum dwellers consume and other eating habits which, needless to add, have a direct beaming on health. Given the intimate link between living environment and health an attempt is made to examine this link.

Table No. 22 - Place of residence

Sl No	Are a	Near Main Road	Per centage	Near Cross Road	Per centage	Near Govt. Office	Per centage	Near Drainage	Per centage	Middle of houses	Per centage	Near Public Toilet	Per centage	Open Space	Per centage
1	B. Nagar	5	10	34	68	0	0	2	4	9	18	0	0	0	0
2	R.G. Nagar	6	12	14	24	0	0	0	0	28	56	2	4	0	0
3	P. Palya	0	0	6	12	0	0	3	6	40	80	1	2	0	0
4	A.J. Nagar	2	4	5	10	0	0	1	2	42	84	0	0	0	0
5	C. Nagar	8	16	12	24	1	2	1	2	28	56	0	0	0	0
All slums		**21**	**8.4**	**71**	**28.4**	**1**	**0.4**	**7**	**2.8**	**147**	**58.8**	**3**	**1.2**	**0**	**0**

From the above table it is clear that though the slums are very much nearer to the main roads, very few house-holds, only 8.4 per cent of the total households are near the main roads. It can also be seen that less than 1 *per cent* households are any where near government office which implies that no government office is situated near the slums. Often it is said that the slums originate either by the side of a big drainage or in the open space available around the drainage but, from the table one can see that very few houses are placed near the drainage. The table also shows the point that there is lack of public toilet facilities in the slums as only 1.2 *per cent* of the house-holds have access to the public toilets. In general, the houses are constructed of poor quality material, since as many as 58.8 per cent of households are surrounded by neighbouring houses with practically little/ no space in between. Living space is one thing that definitely reflects the quality life. Given the cramped extremely congested living space, personal hygiene and genital hygiene are the casualties that render the family members highly vulnerable to sexually related diseases. Owing to limited space, children are exposed to permissive nature of family life and they in turn easily fall prey to unhealthy sexual practices (See the discussions in the preceding pages). They seek to satisfy their quality by actually trying out things out side what they see their parents might be doing at home. Children in slum tend to become sexual deviants and they in turn carry the diseases to people of other sections of society.

Table No: 23 – Living Space

Sl No	Name of the slum	10X10	Per centage	15X10	Per centage	20X20	Per centage	20X15	Per centage	10X30	Per centage	20X30	Per centage	20X10	Per centage
1	B. Nagar	4	8	8	16	19	38	0	0	0	0	19	38	0	0
2	R. Nagar	5	10	25	50	7	14	11	22	1	2	1	2	0	0
3	P. Palya	28	56	19	38	3	6	0	0	0	0	0	0	0	0
4	A. Nagar	2	4	8	16	10	20	6	12	1	2	20	40	3	6
5	C. Nagar	1	2	5	10	7	14	6	12	0	0	24	48	7	14
All slums		40	16	65	26	46	18.4	23	9.2	2	0.8	64	25.6	10	4

It can be seen from the table that 16 per cent of the sample has very small living space of 10X10. 26 per cent of the sample has living space of 15X10 and almost similar per cent i.e. 25.6 per cent has living space of 20X30 which is the highest space. The remaining sample falls in the range as follows: 20X20 (18.4 per cent), 20X15 (9.2 per cent), 30X10 (0.8 per cent) and 20X10 (4 per cent).

Almost half of the sample owns the houses they are living in i.e. 51.6 per cent and the remaining sample i.e. 48.4 per cent are in rented houses.

Table No. 24 - Housing Conditions:								
Sl No	**Name of the Slum**	**Pucca house**	**Per centage**	**Kutcha house**	**Per centage**	**Huts**	**Per centage**	**Total**
1	B. Nagar	38	76	8	16	4	8	50
2	R. Nagar	0	0	41	82	9	18	50
3	P. Palya	3	6	13	26	34	68	50
4	A. Nagar	3	6	16	32	31	62	50
5	C. Nagar	6	12	36	72	8	16	50
All slums		50	20	114	45.6	86	34	250

Housing conditions constitute another important variable. Inadequate housing stock and poor housing conditions create lot of environmental hazards. Poor families often lack the resources that they are unable to avoid situations which might be degrading of their environment. Poor people in crowded squatter settlements frequently endure inadequate access to safe drinking water. Lack of potable safe drinking water forces them to depend upon and overdraw by over-pumping and depletion of ground water. In latest comprehensive large scale sample survey on housing conditions was carried out by NSSO (National Sample Survey Organisation) during January and June 1993. 49th round in both rural and urban area with a sample of 1,19,403 Household, 75,036 from rural sector 44,367 from urban sector. Some of the key results of the survey are as follows:

In the rural sector the share of kutcha, semi-pucca and pucca houses were 32 per cent each respectively whereas in urban sector about 75 per cent Households pucca houses. In the present sample 46 per cent reside in kutcha houses only 20 per cent reside in pucca houses and 34 per cent are in huts. This does not tally with what is reported in the said survey. This would mean that living conditions in slums in Bangalore are very degradable indeed.

Since the living space in their house is already inadequate women who work at residence have to invariably sit in the space available in front of the house which is equally smaller even for proper walking.

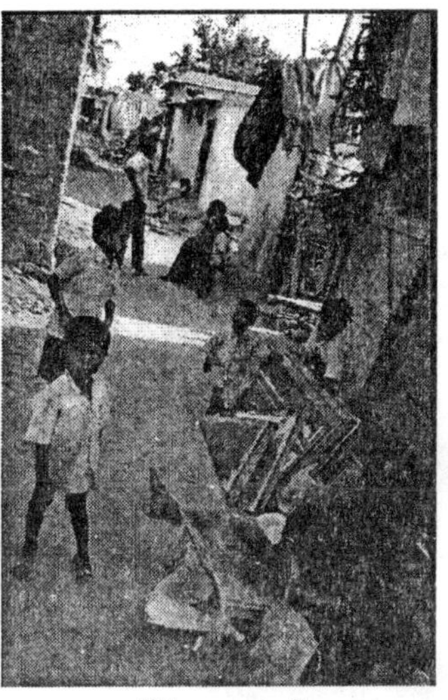

Figure - 9

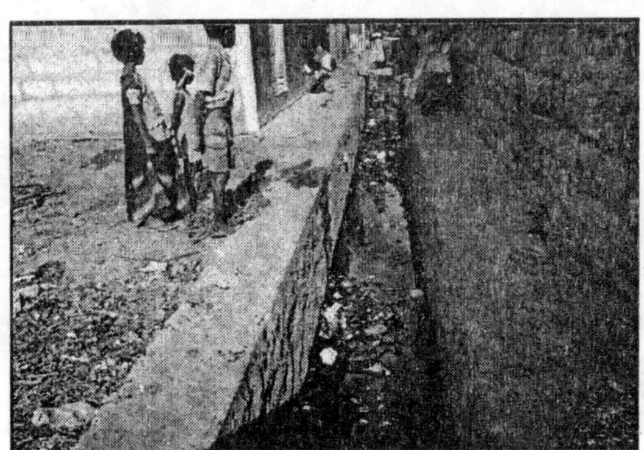

Figure - 10

This photo gives information on the play ground and working place in the slums. The children have to play in front of the house or vacant place near the drainage. The former is alright but the latter is something which is not alright as the area available for playing is not only unhygienic, it is also dangerous. The children may fall in to the gutter; get hurt with broken sharp waste present around; get disease out of infection due to the filth existing; to mention a few.

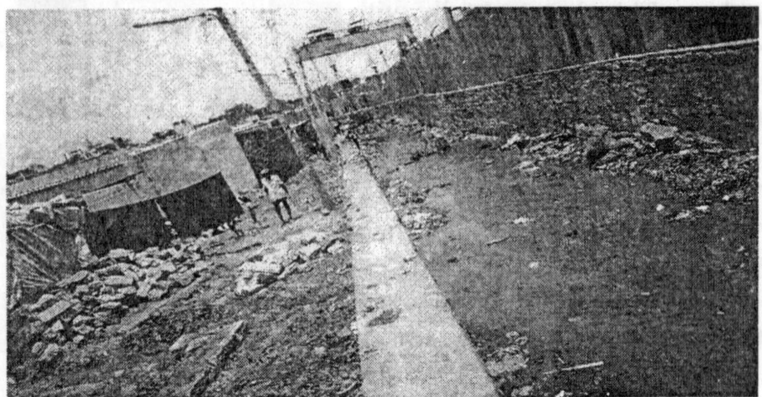

Figure – 11

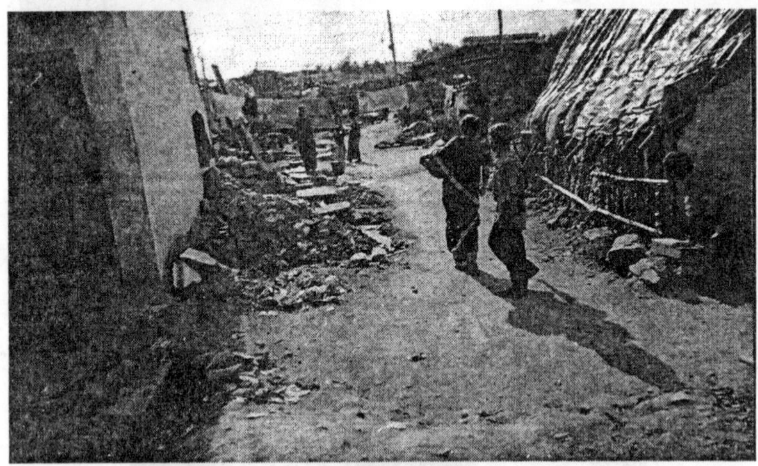

Figure - 12

The above are self explanatory presenting the living environment in the slums. Not to speak of cleanliness, spacious, safe both in terms of health and wealth, basic amenities like drinking water, proper housing, roads etc which are dream words they can never expect under the prevailing situation.

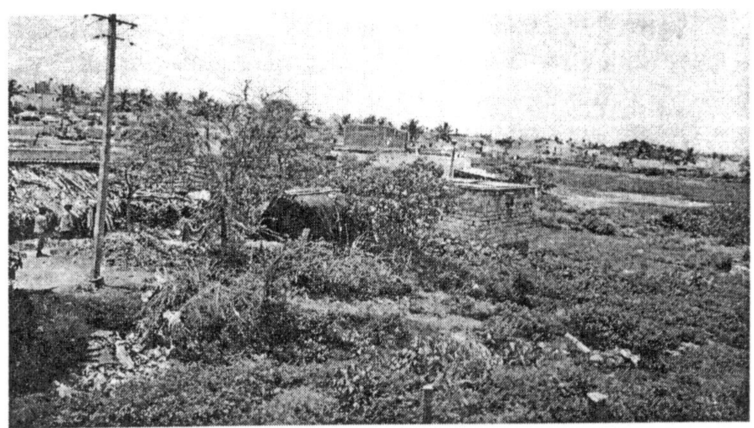

Figure – 13

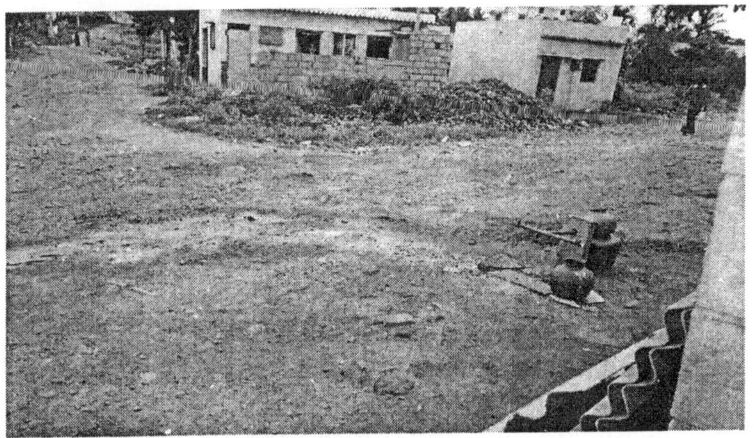

Figure - 14

The above pictures put forth two different conditions; one showing the housing pattern wherein the structure can not even be called a house in one of the older slums and the second showing the housing pattern in one of the upcoming slums. The reason for this may be that though the area is labeled as slum, most of the people who come for living in this area are lower and middle- middle income group people who have struggled a lot to have a house of their own. The water supply existing in the area can also be seen which too speaks of the changing situation. Here we can recall that earlier, in one of the pictures, the area around the water tank is shown where the drainage is passing next to it posing great threat to the health of the users.

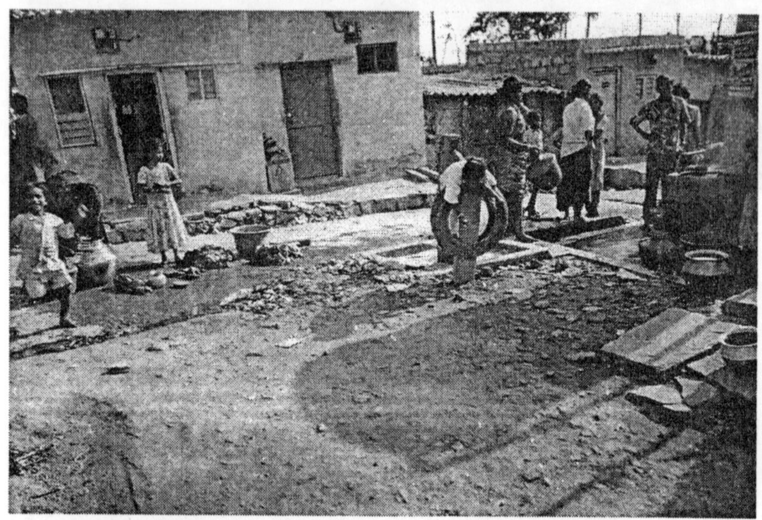

Figure - 15

The above figure shows the environment around the water tank and related activities. It can be seen that the people are washing clothes, children playing and others collecting water in plastic pots and silver utensils for drinking purpose. The other activities carried out around the water tank endanger the purity and safety of the water used for drinking purpose.

This figure throws light on the livelihood of the slum dwellers. It can be seen that a lady is vending vegetables sitting in front of her house which serves as a shop and also as a fruit stall for the residents particularly children who can not afford to buy at big shops in the city. Not to speak of the quality of the fruits as most of he times it would be the rejected or damaged one which has least/no value in the market worth to be thrown into the dustbin. This though serves the purpose, may cause health problems to the consumers especially children.

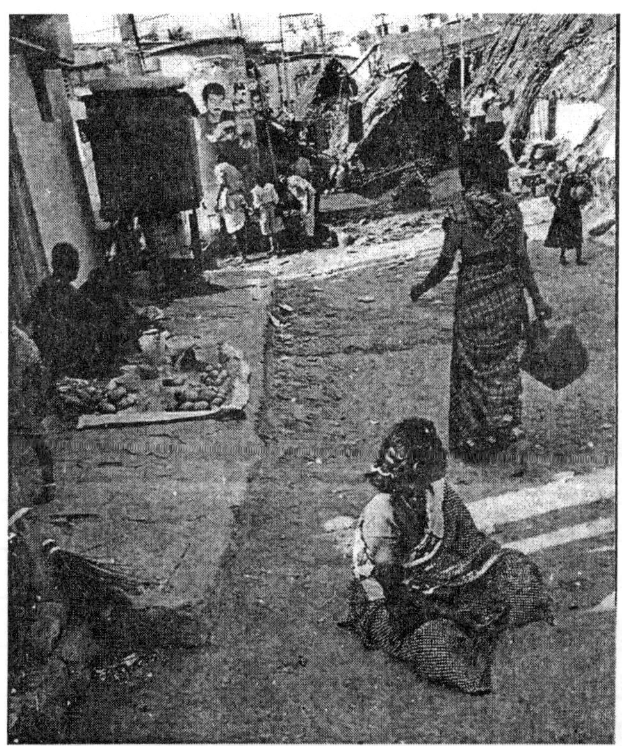

Figure 16

Housing for the millions of homeless people in India has not been a high planning priority. Consequently, at the turn of the century, India will be short of 41 million houses. Can everyone in India be adequately housed? This is one of the hotly debated questions Experience shows no one sector can solve the problems. While the State has failed to meet its primary responsibility of building houses for the poor, the private sector has done little better, building only for profit and for a few.

Inadequate supply: It soon became obvious that the supply of government built low-income housing was hopelessly inadequate in relation to demand. Forced to fend for themselves, the city's poor had no choice but to encroach on vacant plots or footpaths or the strips of land along the railway tracks. They built their own jhopdis, looked out for themselves and managed somehow. Such encroachments were immediately dubbed "illegal", as indeed they were. But where were the poor to go? (Survey of the environment, 1996, housing for urban poor)

Table No. 25- Cooking Energy source

Sl No	Name of the slum	Coal	Per centage	LPG Gas & kerosene.	Per centage	Wood	Per centage	Kerosene.	Per centage	LPG Gas	Per centage
1	B. Nagar	0	0	12	24	0	0	35	70	3	6
2	R. Nagar	0	0	11	22	25	50	11	22	3	6
3	P. Palya	0	0	9	18	4	8	37	74	0	0
4	A. Nagar	0	0	7	14	18	36	24	48	1	2
5	C. Nagar	1	2	18	36	21	42	9	18	1	2
	All slums	1	0.4	57	22.8	68	27.2	116	46.4	8	3.2

By looking into the above table it can be said that, majority of the sample households i.e. 69.2 per cent use kerosene as a main source for cooking. And also it is evident from the table that though the slum residents are usually migrants from rural areas where wood is the main source of energy for cooking, due to non availability of fire wood in the city limits and also because of city impact only 27.2 per cent of the sample is using wood as their source of energy for cooking. This can also be related to the fact that the greenery in and around the city is being reduced to a large extent which is posing a great threat to the city environment in a broader sense. 25.8 per cent of the sample is using LPG for cooking. Though the Government has taken steps to provide the LPG connections, due to poor supply, majority of them depend on Kerosene too in the absence of LPG.

Table No. 26 - Disposal of Waste

Sl No	Name of the Slum	In front of the house	Per centage	Back side of the house	Per centage	Public dust bin	Per centage	Drainage/ Gutter	Per centage	Open space	Per centage	Drainage/ Gutter & Open space	Per centage
1	B. Nagar	5	10	1	2	17	34	7	14	20	40	0	0
2	R. Nagar	0	0	0	0	6	12	0	0	44	88	0	0
3	P. Palya	2	4	0	0	11	22	6	12	30	60	1	2
4	A.J. Nagar	0	0	1	2	10	20	2	4	34	68	3	6
5	C. Nagar	1	2	1	2	8	16	0	0	38	76	2	4
	All slums	8	3.2	3	1.2	52	20.8	15	6	166	66.4	6	2.4

It can be seen from the table that majority of the sample i.e. about 74.4 per cent throw the waste either in open space or gutter. This is the sad state of affair which is affecting the city environment to the maximum extent. The possible reasons for this may be lack of efforts from the Corporation to collect the garbage especially from the slums, lack of infrastructure necessary for the garbage disposal, lack of awareness among the slum people about dangers posed by un-disposed accumulated solid waste.

Table No. 27 - Corporation vehicle for garbage disposal					
Sl No	Name of the Slum	Yes	Per centage	No	Per centage
1	B. Nagar	14	28	36	72
2	R. Nagar	0	0	50	100
3	P. Palya	0	0	50	100
4	A. Nagar	11	22	39	78
5	C. Nagar	0	0	50	100
All slums		25	10	225	90

Though the Corporation is making efforts by launching projects exclusively to improve the garbage disposal called 'Swacha Bengaluru' and 'Nirmala Nagara Yojane' with the involvement of voluntary organisations both in the city limits and also in the CMC areas, still a lot of improvement is needed in this direction, as the table above projects that only two out of five sample slums are getting the Corporation vehicle for garbage collection whereas, the remaining three are devoid of this facility. In those two slums also only 28 per cent and 22 per cent of the people are disposing garbage through the Corporation vehicle which indicates that the coverage is not exhaustive and that the residents are not aware of the advantages of disposing the waste through the vehicle provided by the corporation.

Personal hygiene including genital hygiene is considered a very important factor having a bearing on health. Taking bath is the best way of keeping high personal hygiene. It can be seen from the table that 7.6 per cent of sample take bath everyday though the awareness on the need to maintain personal hygiene seem to be increasing given the danger of spread of infections and sexually transmitted diseases.

Table No. 28 - Hygiene (Personal hygiene taking bath)									
Sl No	Name of the slum	Every day	Per centage	Two days once	Per centage	Weekly twice	Per centage	Weekly once	Per centage
1	B.Nagar	0	0	12	24	36	72	2	4
2	R.Nagar	1	2	23	46	11	22	15	30
3	P.Palya	10	20	29	58	4	8	7	14
4	A.Nagar	8	16	15	30	18	36	9	18
5	C.Nagar	0	0	19	38	16	32	15	30
All slums		19	7.6	98	39.2	85	34	48	19.2

Particularly in the slum this question assumes special significance. Nearly 40 per cent of the sample take bath once in two days, 34 per cent take bath three times in a week. Awareness is there but, due to lack availability of water and lack of facilities to take bath like bath rooms appear to be major constraints. Mere awareness is not sufficient to be able to translate this awareness into actual Behaviours; people require sufficient resources. Given the rapid increase in the size of the slum population, Government often found it increasingly difficult to mobilize sufficient funds to provide all these facilities. The answers to social malady lies in preventing the people migrating from villages to city. There is, therefore an urgent need to promote the development of small towns and medium towns but, also to promote development of villages, to divert funds from the so called city Centreed development activities, to decentralised development activities across the villages.

Table No. 29 - Whether latrine (toilet) facilities available.					
Sl.No	**Latrine (toilet) facilities**	**Yes**	**Per centage**	**No**	**Per centage**
1	B.Nagar	48	96	2	4
2	R.Nagar	36	72	14	28
3	P.Palya	38	76	12	24
4	A.Nagar	48	96	2	4
5	C.Nagar	38	76	12	24
All slums		208	83.2	42	16.8

Table No. 30- If yes Type of latrine (toilet) faciiities available.												
Sl No	**Name of the slum**	**Within the house**	**Per centage**	**Outside the house**	**Per centage**	**Public toilets**	**Per centage**	**Open defecation**	**Per centage**	**Shared latrine**	**Per centage**
1	B. Nagar	2	4	44	88	0	0	2	4	2	4
2	R. Nagar	1	2	34	68	0	0	11	22	4	8
3	P. Palya	1	2	15	30	23	46	11	22	0	0
4	A. Nagar	1	2	14	28	33	66	2	4	0	0
5	C. Nagar	1	2	33	66	4	8	12	24	0	0
All slums		6	2.4	140	56	60	24	38	15.2	6	2.4

From the point view of clean environment, community hygiene, family hygiene, and personal hygiene, toilet and bath room facilities play a very important role. In several slums due to lack of latrine facilities slum people defecate in open air and majority children do so. In areas very close to slums, people living in neighborhood having felt the heat of environmental degradation due to open deification government and non-governmental organisations have been extending benefits of toilet facilities to slums. This is evident from the table. 83.2 per cent of sample reported to have toilet facilities. A total of 58.4 per cent of them have individual toilets and out of the remaining, 24 per cent of them use public toilets besides 2.4 per cent of shared latrine users and 15.2 per cent are open defecators.

The central government has given acceptance for the construction of 1000 toilets in the slums of Karnataka under "Nirmala Bharath Abhiyana". Out of 1000,500 will be with in Bangalore slums. Under Vambe and NIrmala Jyothi Projects, 33,000 houses will be constructed for the slum dwellers.

Table No. 31 - Drinking water availability

Sl No	Name of the slum	With in the house	Per centage	Out side the house	Per centage
1	B. Nagar	9	18	41	82
2	R. Nagar	1	2	49	98
3	P. Palya	0	0	50	100
4	A. Nagar	0	0	50	100
5	C. Nagar	0	0	50	100
All slums		10	4	240	96

Another variable which could reflect the health condition of people is safe drinking water. It is reported that 90 per cent of the sample draw water from community taps. It is only in case of Bapuji Nagar slum as already noted earlier as developed slum, 18 per cent reported to possess individual home based taps. This clearly indicates that there is still lack of basic amenities in slums. Lake of individual taps is due to the non-availability of sufficient safe drinking water. Given the depletion of underground water, irregular rains, the picture is becoming increasingly precarious.

Table No. 32 - Water source														
Sl No	Name of the Slum	Indl.Tap	Per centage	Indl. Hand pump	Per centage	Indl. Well	Per centage	Comm. Tap	Per centage	Comm. Hand pump	Per centage	Comm. Well	Per centage
1	B. Nagar	9	18	0	0	0	0	41	82	0	0	0	0
2	R. Nagar	0	0	0	0	1	4	48	96	1	2	0	0
3	P. Palya	0	0	0	0	0	0	45	90	1	2	4	8
4	A. Nagar	0	0	0	0	0	0	47	94	2	4	1	2
5	C. Nagar	2	4	3	6	0	0	43	86	1	2	1	2
All slums		11	4.4	3	1.2	1	0.4	224	89.6	5	2	6	2.4

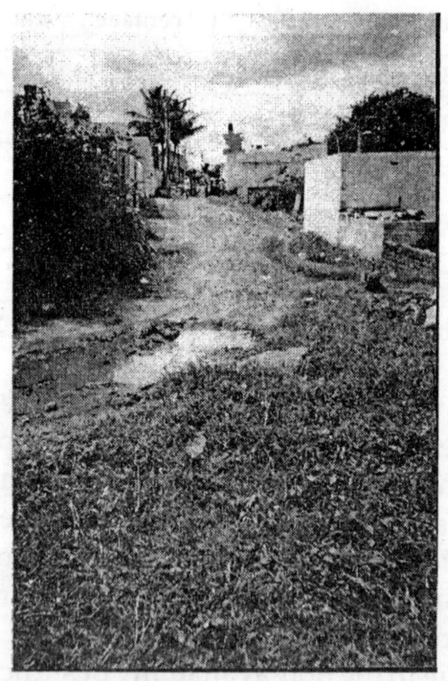

Figure - 18

Only 4.4 per cent of the total sample is able to possess individual home based taps which shows the poor accessibility of the facilities by the respondents and also their inability to avail the existing facilities. Another reason for this could be lack of space for having taps inside the house, as the living space available is very little and inadequate even for proper accommodation.

3.2 per cent of hand pumps are there including 2 per centof common and 1.2 per cent of individual pumps. The depletion of ground water level drastically in the last decade may be attributed for less number of hand pumps along with high cost factor involved in getting an individual hand pump through digging of bore-well.

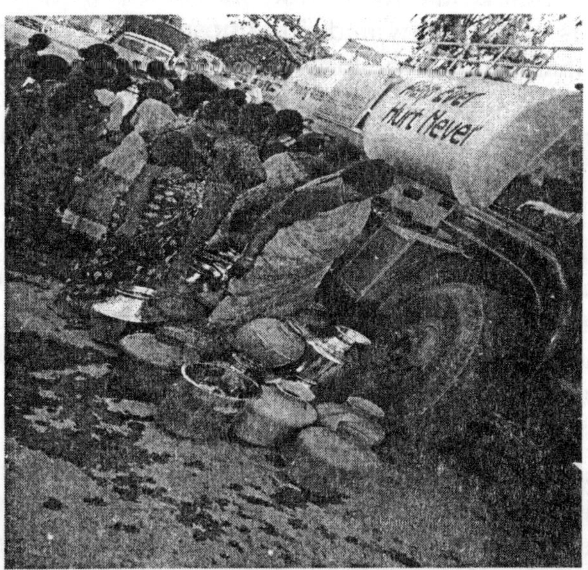

Figure - 18

The roads in the slums are captured in this wherein one can see that even in upcoming slums roads are still mud ones and during rainy seasons the potholes fill up with water proving dangerous to both pedestrians and riders.

The other picture shows the difficulty faced in getting water for drinking where the Corporation has provided neither the tanks nor the taps.

DRINKING WATER AND SANITATION:

Inadequate sanitation is a major cause of the degradation of the quality of the ground water and surface water. Sanitation is closely linked with infant mortality rate and life expectancy. The infant mortality rate in developed countries of the world is 8 per thousand live-births as against 62 in developing countries in the world. Inadequate facilities for disposal of garbage lead to large scale quantity of waste going into both ground water and surface water. Ground water contamination is less visible but often more serious. Smoke and fumes from indoor use of bio-mass fuel such as wood, straw and dung pose much greater health risks than outdoor pollution. Women and children suffer most from this from of pollution. Its effect on health is equivalent to those of smoking several packs of cigarettes a day.

An all India survey on conditions of drinking water, sanitation and hygiene prevailing during the period January-June 1998 was carried out as part of the 54th round of the NSSO. This survey is the only nationwide enquiry to provide estimates on certain characteristics of availability and use or drinking water and on some conditions of sanitation and hygiene at the national level.

The sample design adopted for the survey was a stratified multi-stage for both rural and urban. The census villages and urban frame survey blocks were the first stage units (FSU's) for the rural and urban sectors respectively. Households were the ultimate stage sampling units in both the sectors. The numbers of villages and UFS blocks surveyed were 5,115 and 1,745 respectively. The actual number of households surveyed was 78,990 in the rural sector and 31,323 in the urban sector.

DRINKING WATER:

An estimated 50 per cent of rural households were served by tube well/hand pump while an estimated 26 per cent and 19 per cent were served by well and tap respectively. About 70 per cent and 21 per cent of urban households are being served by tap and tube well/hand pump respectively. About 18 per cent households in both rural and urban areas are using some supplementary source of drinking water. Tube-well hand pump was the most frequently used supplementary source. In rural areas about 18 per cent of households reported to have filtered their drinking water but very few households reported to have chemically treated or boiled water before drinking. The situation was slightly better in urban areas where the *per cent*age of households reporting boiling and filtering of drinking water before consumption were 11 per cent and 35 per cent respectively.

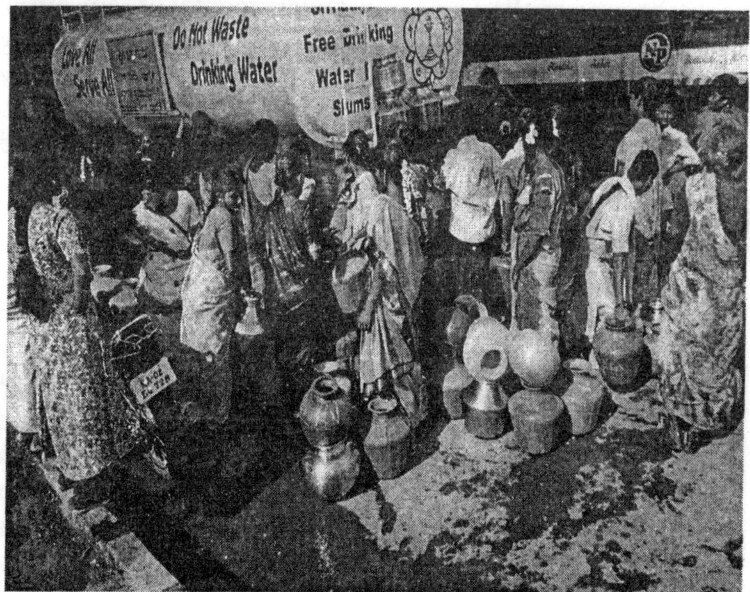

Figure - 19

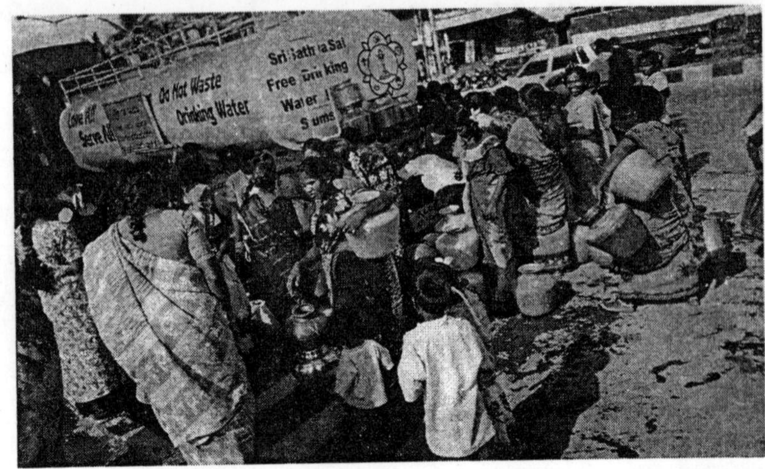

Figure - 20

The above pictures unveil the problem of drinking water prevailing in slums. The residents have to depend on tank water being supplied by a non-governmental organisation. There is no water supply in the slum in spite of it being situated very next to the highway road. This being the situation of a well established slum, it left to the readers to imagine the conditions in other remote and unaddressed slums in the city.

SANITATION:

The proportion of households reporting no bathroom was much higher in rural areas (81 per cent) than that in urban areas (35 per cent). As high as 83 per cent of households, in rural areas reported using no latrine, as against only 26 per cent in urban areas. Further only about 8 per cent and 1 per cent of rural households reported using septic tank and sewerage system compared to 35 per cent and 22 per cent of urban households. The proportion of households reporting removal of household waste by household members was much higher (94 per cent) in rural areas than that (71 per cent) in urban areas. while 14 per cent and 12 per cent of urban households reported removal of their waste by local authorities and by private arrangement among residents respectively. the corresponding *per cent*ages were almost negligible in rural areas. about 2/3rds (67 per cent) of rural households and less than 30 per cent of urban households reported their waste being taken to individual dumping spots. While a substantial *per cent*age (47 per cent) of urban households reported removal of their waste community dumping spot, only 4 per cent of rural households reported the same. The estimates of poverty have been released from the year 1973-74 onwards using the full survey data on household consumption expenditure collected by the NSSO. The results show that during the last two decades the per centage of population below poverty line has declined significantly in rural areas as well as in urban areas, but still after 50 years of independence India is facing an acute problem of poverty.

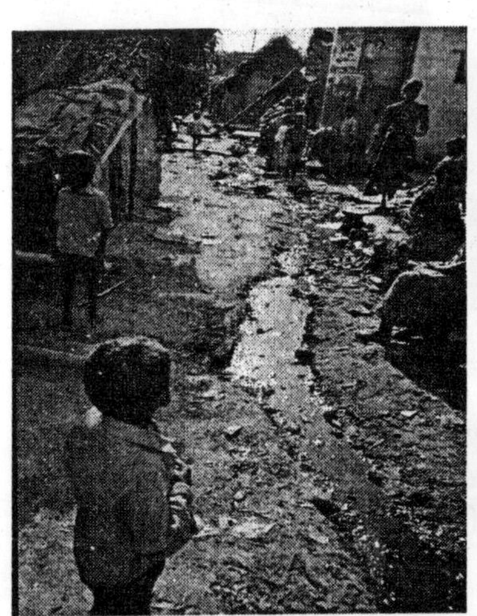

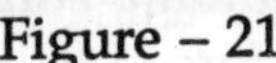

Figure – 21

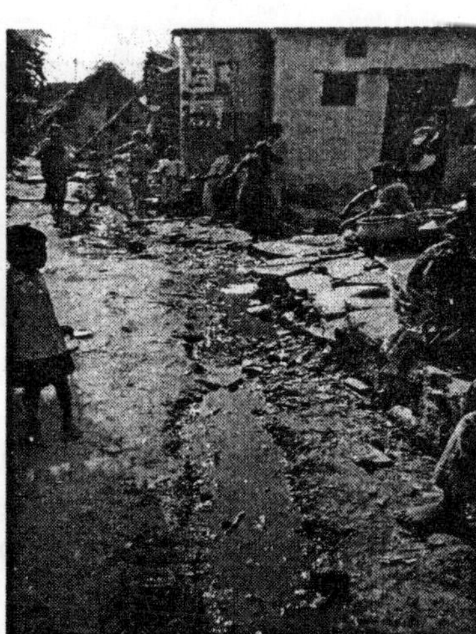

Figure – 22

The pictures depict the sorry state of affairs with regards to cleanliness and hygiene of the living environment. Another eye catchy point note worthy here is the existence of mini water tank meant for drinking water supply. One can clearly see women collecting water from the tank for drinking purpose. From this only one can guess about the serious health hazards which people suffer sue to the manner in which water is collected stored and used. Given thus unclean environment slum people in general and elderly and children in particular get exposed to and suffer from a wide-range of health hazards.

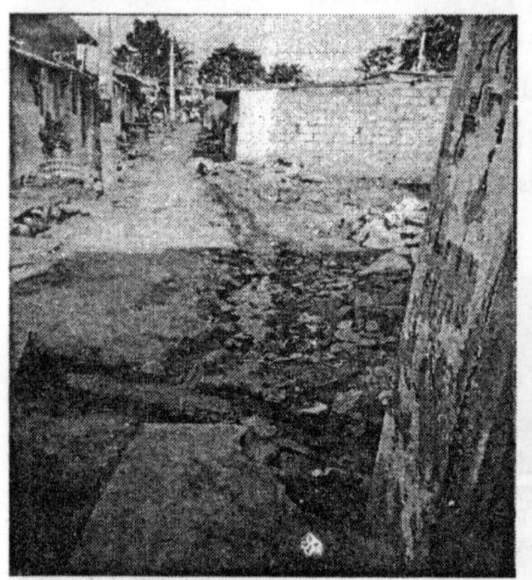

Figure – 23

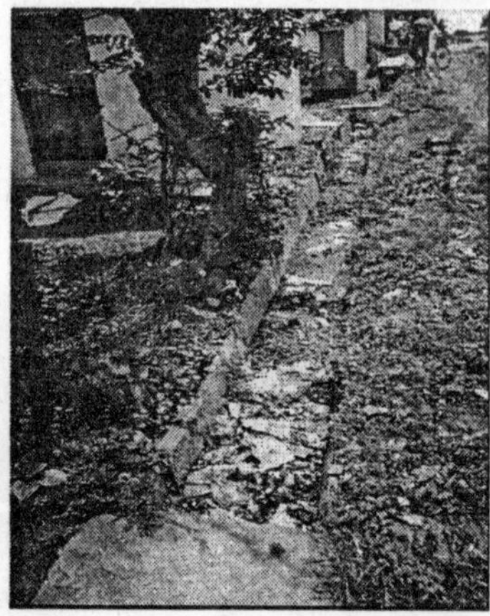

Figure – 24

The above picture throws light on the existing drainage system in the slum. One can see that it is open and running in front of the house with lot of filth in it leading to a number of health risks.

In this picture we can see an open drainage running in between two lanes of houses. People are forced to live with this. The houses being constructed by the Corporation, do not give adequate attention to safety and sanitary condition.

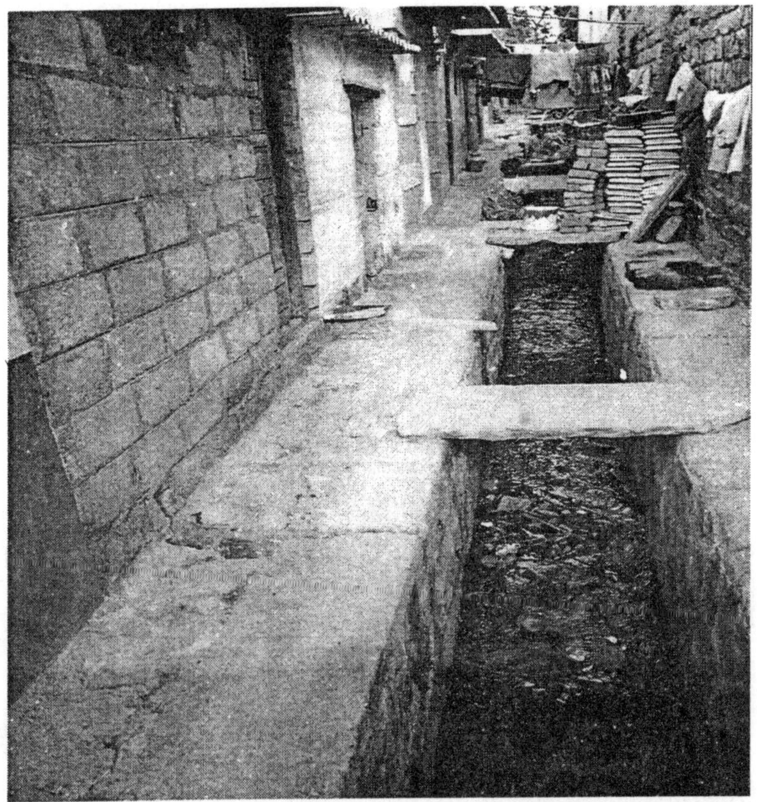

Figure - 25

Open drains are not only dangerous to children but become breeding place for mosquitoes, pigs and street dogs which often spread the diseases.

The women are engaged in their daily household chores on the drainage itself. Even the children are inevitably made to play there. Let with no alternative even children are forced to play over these which playing children might fall in to the drainage thus risking their life.

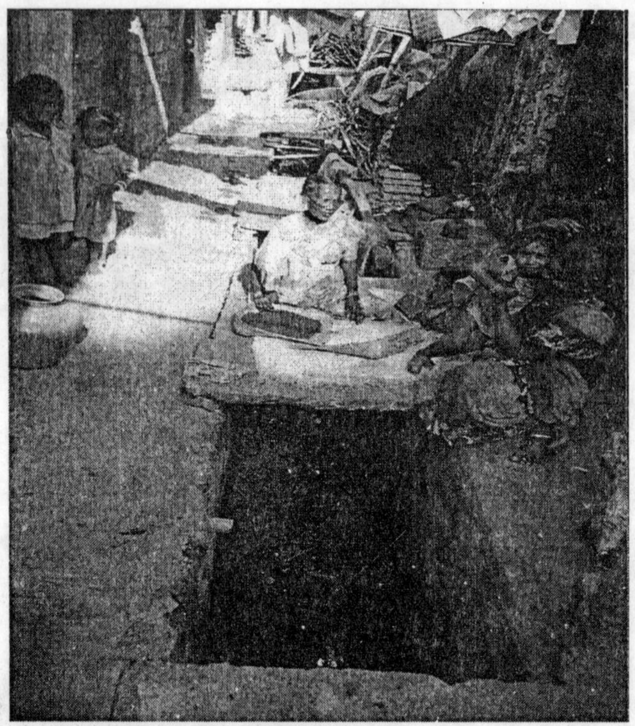

Figure – 26

In continuation of the above, these pictures try to substantiate the above said by capturing the boys playing very next to the drainage passing along. It also throws some light on the condition of the drainage as well. It can be seen that the drainage has silted up with lot of garbage and needs to be cleaned up. Otherwise, it would become the major cause for health hazards which pose a great threat to the health conditions of the dwellers around. It can also we seen that the place is also being used for open defection which adds up to the health hazards.

From the table one can see the prevailing sanitary conditions in the slums. It is very shocking to see that in spite of efforts put in by the Government to provide proper sanitary

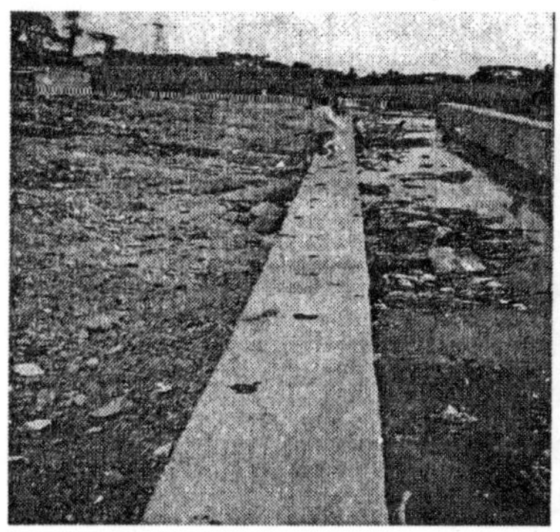

Figure – 27

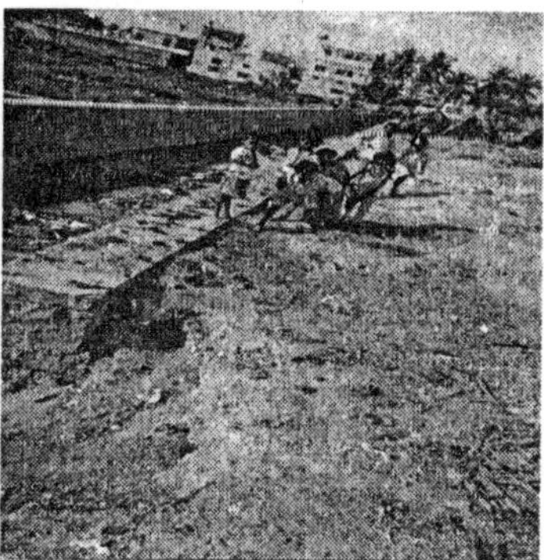

Figure - 28

Table No 33 - Sanitary facilities

Sl. No.	Name of the Slum	yes	Per centage	No	Per centage
1	B. Nagar	0	0	50	100
2	R. Nagar	0	0	50	100
3	P. Palya	0	0	50	100
4	A. Nagar	28	56	22	44
5	C. Nagar	4	8	46	92
	All slums	32	12.8	218	87.2

Table No 34 - Pattern of sanitary

Sl. No	Name of the Slum	Open	Per centage	Close	Per centage	Not applicable	Per centage
1	B. Nagar	0	0	0	0	50	100
2	R. Nagar	0	0	0	0	50	100
3	P. Palya	0	0	0	0	50	100
4	A. Nagar	10	20	18	36	22	44
5	C. Nagar	2	4	2	4	46	92
	All slums	12	4.8	20	8	218	87.2

facilities to the public in the city, a very little has been done in this direction with regard to slums. Greater effort both by government and non government organisation are needed. The table reveals that there exists no sanitary facilities as such in three of the sample slums and in the other two where it is said to be existing is more nominal in nature than functional as only a total of 12.8 per centof the sample are said to have these facilities out of which, 4.8 per cent are open drainages and 8 per centare of closed type. As already discussed, these factors are much contributory in making slums vulnerable to diseases and also eco-dangerous in nature.

MIGRATION

It is widely reported that increase in the size of the slum population has been due to rural urban migration. The so called "push factors" like poverty, unemployment, loss of sources of lively hood due to natural calamities like famine, floods and drought make large number of people of almost all age groups except very old and invalid people to migrate to the cities in search of lively-hood. Such people when they reach city try to find shelter in slums or create a slum on vacant lands.

Table No. 35 - Migration Profile

Sl No	Name of the slum	With in the district (localities)	Per centag e	Out side the district/wit hin the state	Per centage	Out side the state	Per centag e
1	B. Nagar	32	64	6	12	12	24
2	R. Nagar	37	74	4	8	9	18
3	P. Palya	39	78	1	2	10	20
4	A, Nagar	33	66	7	14	10	20
5	C. Nagar	40	80	2	4	8	16
All slums		181	72	20	8	49	20

Of the sample, 72.4 per cent are migrants though apparently they reported to have come from villages with in the districts and 19.6 per cent of the sample reported to have come from out side the state. Bangalore city geographically located close to other neighbor states of Tamil Nadu and Andhra Pradesh and compared to the other parts of the state like hence a proportion of the samples are migrants from out side the state. Only 8 per cent of the sample reported to have come from out side districts but with in the state. Among other things, the data reiterates the fact that increase in size of the slum population and increasing number of slums have been due to rural urban migration. Urban poverty is thus an out growth of rural poverty. Urban poor are highly vulnerable and they pose serious challenges to urban environment. Unwieldy and uncontrollable slum population has been threat to clean environment. A study conducted on slum people and urban poor reported that the *per cent*age of immigrants ranged from 70 to 90 *per cent*. An immigrant refers to those households whose lead was born in another place that the present one in the slum or community (Sunikumar Karn and Others, 2003)

Table No. 36 - Disease burden in slums April 2004 to March 2005

Sl. No	Month	Number of persons seeking treatment	Type of Diseases										Total
			Fever/ abdomen pain/ headache	Per centage	Diarrhea/ Vomiting	Per centage	Anti Natal Care	Per centage	Dog bite	Per centage	Others	Per centage	
1	April	279	28	10.0358	24	8.602151	24	8.602	18	6.45	185	66.308	279
2	May	521	38	7.29367	26	4.990403	28	5.374	20	3.84	409	78.503	521
3	June	490	50	10.2041	31	6.326531	46	9.388	20	4.08	343	70	490
4	July	373	31	8.31099	14	3.753351	24	6.434	25	6.7	279	74.799	373
5	August	439	29	6.60592	35	7.972665	52	11.85	18	4.1	305	69.476	439
6	September	465	30	6.45161	30	6.451613	63	13.55	24	5.16	318	68.387	465
7	October	315	26	8.25397	25	7.936508	44	13.97	29	9.21	191	60.635	315
8	November	311	27	8.68167	26	8.360129	38	12.22	26	8.36	194	62.379	311
9	December	325	24	7.38462	23	7.076923	31	9.538	23	7.08	224	68.923	325
10	January	412	39	9.46602	26	6.31068	40	9.709	48	11.7	259	62.864	412
11	February	531	36	6.77966	25	4.708098	42	7.91	32	6.03	396	74.576	531
12	March	487	33	6.77618	22	4.517454	40	8.214	30	6.16	362	74.333	487
13	Total	4948	391	7.90218	307	6.204527	472	9.539	313	6.33	3465	70.028	4948

This table describes about various types of diseases that occur among the slum dwellers. This information is pertaining to Pantharapalya slum wherein, a Corporation Hospital is present. This hospital is exclusively meant for Reproductive Child Health programme through which it provides the services of maternal and child health care. Apart from these, it also takes care of general health needs of the local residents.

From the table one can see the total number of patients availing treatment month-wise. Apart from common day-to-day problems like fever, head ache, etc. problems like gastritis, arthritis. etc, is increasingly becoming common amongst others. This may be attributed to changing life styles and working conditions in the city environment. Diarrhea/vomiting and Dog bite seem to more common. Inadequate supply of potable and safe drinking water, nutritious food and unhygienic living conditions being the reason for the former, latter may be due to lack of efforts by the Corporation to curtail the population of road side dogs, lack of space for playing, densely populated houses and narrow roads could also make the children more vulnerable to dog bites.

Reference

1. Egberttellegen and Maarten Wolsink, University of Amsterdam. Netherlands 1994: *Society - Its Environment*, Gordon and Breach Science Publishers.
2. *Human Development Report*, 1997, the United Nations Development Programme
3. Statistics from Pantharapalya Health Centre - April 2004 to March 2005.
4. Kumar, Sunil, Snigeo Shikura, Hideki Harada, (2003): *Living Environment and Health of Urban Poor*, journal: Economic and political weekly, Vol:6 No.Aug-2003. Samiksha Trust publication.

CHAPTER V

ENVIRONMENTAL CONSCIOUSNESS: AN EMPIRICAL ANALYSIS

Perception, attitude and values among other things, together determine human personality. An analysis of these aspects of the sample of slum population becomes absolutely essential for assessing the role of human Behaviours in the field of environmental protection and environmental management. Unfortunately, the whole question of environmental management has almost invariably been entrusted to formal institutions like some slum clearance boards, city municipal corporation, urban development authorities and pollution control boards etc, not to speck of a wide variety of non-governmental voluntary agencies who claim to play a very important role in improving the environmental conditions of slum people in particular and urban residents in general. Given the ostensibly government character and semi government character of these organisations, the quality of service rendered by these organisations is very poor due to so called problems of bureaucracy like corruption, delay in implementation, lack of quality in the inputs provided. In the entire exercise people are not involved and naturally not only people tend to develop what is called 'dependency syndrome' but also they become increasingly reluctant to initiate concerted collective action for a common cause. In this context, development theories, environmental activists have pleaded for the involvement of the local people not only in the management of common property resources but also in the management of local environments. Local population both individually as well as collectively has been found responsible for lot of environmental changes. Most environmental changes that have hither to occurred have been largely negative and hence these changes have come to pose serious and grave health risks, but also fast depletion of life-support resources. In order to encourage people to participate positively, the quality of human material must improve, As it is, slum population can not be expected to be sensitive to environmental concerns. They need to be educated, motivated, mobilised and organised if necessary trained for a planned, consolidated, collective action. Before attempt is made to embark (venture) up on this task, it is necessary to study and empirically ascertain the type and quality of slum population. There are a lot of myths misunderstandings regarding slum people. Our attitude towards them is influenced by stereotypes and one is not very sure of them unless sound knowledge is obtained of them by means of serious empirical social research. Apart from the social background which we discussed in the previous chapter; an attempt is made to discover the human personality of slum people on the basis of empirical analysis of perception, attitude, values and knowledge of the sample of slum population is regard to environmental changes.

Understanding how a community perceives health risks apparently caused by as polluted water, inadequate drainage, or lack of garbage collection is essential to designing effective programmes to address these problems. Individuals perceive risks to their health through a lens derived from their cultural, economic, societal, and educational backgrounds and respond accordingly. For example, a squatter in a slum in Calcutta, might happily boil water collected at a public tap rather than move to a house with piped water that was located far from job opportunities; a middleclass family in Los Angeles would probably make a very different choice. Until recently, these differences in how people view and respond to risks were not part of formal health risk analysis, which has traditionally relied on statistical correlations between exposure to risks and the incidence of various illnesses. Now, health planners are beginning to realize that using such objective measures of risk to design public health projects without accounting for how the affected community itself views the health risk being addressed is a cause for failure public health programmes. Residents of the slums are well aware of the health risks associated with fire accidents floods and contamination of water although they might not know the epidemiological details of pollution and contamination. They are all too familiar with the symptoms that they suffer. Can risks to health from environmental hazards be reduced in a way that integrates community perceptions and priorities? Some recent efforts to address the health problems surrounding solid waste collections prove that this approach can succeed. Although the formal urban planner considers municipal garbage a health and environmental hazard, many of the poor who earn their livings as scavengers look upon urban waste as an economic resource from which marketable products can be derived. In cities throughout the developing world, scavengers collect waste such as plastic, paper, glass, tin cans, and bones, contributing greatly to garbage collection and recycling efforts in the city. Of course, scavenging is hazardous employment. It is poverty driven, undertaken by the most vulnerable people - often women and children. In the process of sorting through trash, scavengers expose themselves to serious health hazards such as injuries from broken glass and cans and are disproportionately exposed to disease-carrying pests that breed in garbage. *(The Urban Environment, World Resources – 1996-97)*

Table-No. 37 - Self perception of motive regarding marital relation													
Sl No	**Name of theSlum**	**Excellent**	**Per centage**	**Very good**	**Per centage**	**Good**	**Per centage**	**Not bad**	**Per centage**	**Bad**	**Per centage**	**Unmarried**	**Per centage**
1	**B. Nagar**	1	2	22	44	27	54	0	0	0	0	0	0
2	**R. Nagar**	3	6	11	22	36	72	0	0	0	0	0	0
3	**P. Palya**	0	0	7	14	43	86	0	0	0	0	0	0
4	**A. Nagar**	0	0	6	12	43	86	0	0	0	0	1	2
5	**C. Nagar**	1	2	26	52	22	44	0	0	0	0	1	2
	All slums	5	2	72	28.8	171	68.4	0	0	0	0	2	0.8

Self perception about marital relation plays an important role in one's life. It is very much necessary to know what one thinks about the marital relationship and also his feelings towards it. It enables us to assess the relationship between husband and wife and also the quality of life being led by them. If the perception is very good or good it implies that the person is happy with his family relationships and this leads to betterment in quality and satisfaction in life. As it can be seen from the table, the entire samples which are married are of the opinion that their marital relations are either very good or good in nature and thus their perceptions too are similar. This shows that whether it is love marriage or arranged marriage, in India in general and Hindus in particular opine that marriage is a bond which is a God's gift and is made in heaven and thus, one should carry it through out their life and it continues to their next life also. Because of this, there are very few Divorce cases among Indians when compared to Western Societies even though the number of cases has gone up in recent years because of degradation of our values and norms by the younger generations due to the impact of western culture and also the increased torture on women by men due to superiority complex of male domination in the society.

Table-No. 38 - Self-perception regarding intercourse.

Sl No	Name of the slum	Bear children	Per centage	Entertainment	Per centage	Bear children & Religious (consideration)	Per centage	Bear children and entertainment	Per centage	Bear children, Entertainment & Religious (consideration)	Per centage
1	B. Nagar	11	22	3	6	3	6	28	56	5	10
2	R. Nagar	30	60	9	18	5	10	6	12	0	0
3	P.Palya	33	60	2	18	2	10	0	0	13	26
4	A. Nagar	27	54	3	6	1	2	19	38	0	0
5	C. Nagar	17	34	1	2	0	0	32	64	0	0
All Slums		118	47.2	18	7.2	11	4.4	85	34	18	7.2

With the above background one can say that in our society, marriage is a relationship which has many good reasons to state than mere entertainment i.e., physical enjoyment. It is considered as a religious ritual to be performed by every men and women in order to meet the religious requirements. In 'Vedas' it is clearly stated that any person must follow the Four Ashramas, Brahmacharya, Grihastha, Vanaprastha and Sanyasa in his course of life. In Grihasthashrama one has to get married and beget children for procreation and also salvation from his life through the male children. Thus, marriage as said above is important as a religious ritual. Though in the present society religion has lost the importance it had earlier, even today it plays a considerable role in one's life and hence as many as 11.6

per cent put together are of the opinion that intercourse has religious consideration. The table shows that bearing children is assumed to be the most important reason for intercourse as 47.2 per cent has replied so. Only a small *per cent* i.e., about 7.2 have replied that it is for entertainment purpose.

Table-No. 39 - Attitude towards sex

Sl No	Name of the slum	Permissive & Value based	Per centage	Restrictions	Per centage	Value based	Per centage	Restrictions & Value based	Per centage	Permissive	Per centage	D.K	Per centage
1	B.Nagar	6	12	14	28	16	32	14	28	0	0	0	0
2	R.Nagar	1	2	35	70	14	28	0	0	0	0	0	0
3	P.Palya	2	4	34	68	12	24	2	4	0	0	0	0
4	A.Nagar	0	0	36	72	8	16	5	10	0	0	1	2
5	C.Nagar	1	2	14	28	12	24	20	40	2	4	1	2
	All slums	10	4	133	53.2	62	24.8	41	16.4	2	0.8	2	0.8

Among the sample surveyed, when enquired about their attitude towards sex, more than half of the sample i.e., 53.2 per cent answered that there are restrictions on this. This has direct relation with our social environment which has put restrictions on even open discussions about sex and related topics. We have been brought up in a situation where, thinking about sex or talking on it in front of the family members itself is considered as an offence. It is looked at as purely personal and confidential issue between the partners and is not to be discussed in front of others. Hence, the people are of the opinion that there are restrictions on sex and related issues and should not be deliberated in an open Dias. It is more of a value based issue as in our sacred books sex is considered as a duty to be performed by the married couple to beget children in order to procreate and continue their generation and to get 'Moksha' after their death through the children, especially male. Hence, it is more of value based rather than physical desire to us which has influenced the answers of our sample. 24.8 per cent of them have said that it is value based and 16.4 per cent have said it to be both restrictive and value based. The remaining are of the opinion that it is permissive and few of them also say that it is value based.

Table-No. 40 - Contraction of diseases.

Sl No	Name of the slum	Husband	Per centage	Wife	Per centage	Those who have multiple sex partners	Per centage	Not applicable	Per centage	D.K	Per centage
1	B. Nagar	0	0	0	0	14	28	36	72	0	0
2	R. Nagar	0	0	0	0	34	70	16	26	0	0
3	P. Palya	0	0	0	0	26	52	24	48	0	0
4	A. Nagar	0	0	0	0	21	42	29	58	0	0
5	C. Nagar	0	0	0	0	22	44	27	54	1	2
All slums		0	0	0	0	117	46.8	132	52.8	1	0.4

Among 46.8 per cent of those who know about the occurrence of these types of diseases, all are of the opinion that it comes to only those who have multiple sex partners. The remaining sample is unaware or is not competent enough to understand these types of diseases which pose a great threat to their well being. It shows the poor level of awareness among them which is mainly responsible for the occurrence of such diseases in them much severely than in their counterparts.

Table-No. 41 - Treatment seeking behaviour

Sl No	Name of the slum	Govt. Hospital	Per centage	Pvt.& govt Hospitals	Per centage	Ayurvedic Hospital	Per centage	Local Hospitals	Per centage	Mantra, tayata	Per centage	Not Applicable	Per centage	Don't now	Per centage	Others	Per centage
1	B. Nagar	5	10	9	18	0	0	0	0	0	0	36	72	0	0	0	0
2	R. Nagar	16	32	17	34	0	0	0	0	0	0	16	32	1	2	0	0
3	P. Palya	0	0	1	2	0	0	0	0	0	0	24	48	2	4	23	46
4	A. Nagar	9	10	1	18	4	8	1	2	0	0	30	72	5	10	0	0
5	C. Nagar	5	10	9	18	0	0	0	0	0	0	28	56	8	16	0	0
All Slums		35	14	37	14.8	4	1.6	1	0.4	0	0	134	54	16	6.4	23	9.2

This question was mainly asked with an intention to assess the attitude of the sample population with regard to diseases in general and these type of diseases in particular which are looked upon differently. If a person is said to have this type of disease, his character is looked down upon by the society and he is treated as an untouchable in most of the cases. Hence, people though suffering from any of these kinds of diseases dare not to disclose and even try to hide it from the eyes of the family members unless is takes serious turns. They even hesitate to go to the Doctor and try to get treatment confidentially through some half-trained or some illegal practitioner, or a person who gives local medicines made out of some tree extracts like leaves, roots, bark, fruits, etc. Apart from this, lack of access to treatment and medicines is another reason for them to go with what is locally available.

Table-No. 42 – Do you know about sexually transmitted infection/diseases					
Sl No	Name of the slum	Yes	Per centage	No	Per centage
1	B. Nagar	12	24	38	76
2	R. Nagar	31	62	19	38
3	P. Palya	26	52	24	48
4	A. Nagar	20	40	30	60
5	C. Nagar	22	44	28	56
All slums		111	44.4	139	55.6

Table-No. 43 - Knowledge of disease and sex					
Sl No	Name of the slum	Yes	Per centage	No	Per centage
1	B. Nagar	16	32	34	68
2	R. Nagar	32	64	18	36
3	P. Palya	26	52	24	48
4	A. Nagar	21	42	29	58
5	C. Nagar	22	44	28	56
All slums		117	46.8	133	53.2

This question was basically asked to assess the basic knowledge of the slum people on various aspects related to health, particularly on the diseases which are related to sexual behaviour among them. It is normally said that the slum people have deviant Behavioural attitudes; they do not follow the regular norms and values existing in the society. Similarly they are said to act according to their whims and fancies with regard to sex too. It is generally observed that the slum people are not aware of sexually transmitted diseases and its severity due to lack of awareness and also understanding capacity. Lack of personal hygiene and early marriage leading to early beginning of sexual activities seem to be the major cause for STDs to occur among slum people. Women are more prone to these types of diseases as they are bodily weak and also lack proper guidance to avoid such problems. As a result of the efforts made by the Government and non-governmental organisations to provide awareness to the slum people regarding these types of diseases, it can be seen from the tables that about 44.4 per cent and 46.8 per cent of them are aware of the occurrence of these types of diseases. In spite of this, it also becomes important to note that the remaining 55.6 per cent and 55.2 per cent of them are still unaware about these things which imply that a lot more is pending to be done in this direction.

Table-No. 44 - Awareness on sexually transmitted infections and diseases. (STIs/STDs)

Sl No	Name of the slum	Aids	Per centage	Gajji	Per centage	Hunnu	Per centage	Cancer	Per centage	No response	Per centage	Infections	Per centage	D.K	Per centage
1	B. Nagar	7	14	1	2	3	6	0	0	35	70	0	0	4	8
2	R. Nagar	23	46	0	0	0	0	1	2	26	52	0	0	0	0
3	P. Palya	25	50	0	0	0	0	1	2	24	48	0	0	0	0
4	A. Nagar	16	32	0	0	1	2	2	4	29	58	1	2	1	2
5	C. Nagar	18	36	1	2	1	2	2	4	28	56	0	0	0	0
All slums		89	35.6	2	0.8	5	2	6	2.4	142	56.8	1	0.4	5	2

The above table further supports the ignorance of the slum dwellers about Sexually Transmitted Diseases and Infections. They are even poor in identifying the type of disease which is troubling them. Because of the importance given to HIV/AIDS 35.6 per cent of them are of the opinion that any sex related disease could be named as HIV/AIDS. 56.8 per cent of them are unaware of STDs/STIs. Out of the remaining, 3.6 per cent of them opine that it may be Gajji, Hunnu or infection. Most of these diseases occur due to unhygienic and unhealthy living conditions prevailing in slums. Even cleanliness also contributes for this. In fact personal hygiene in general and genital hygiene in particular goes a long way in reducing the vulnerability for these diseases.

Table-No. 45 - Contraction of diseases

Sl No	Name of the slum	Yes	Per centage	No	Per centage	No Response	Per centage
1	B. Nagar	14	28	36	72	0	0
2	R. Nagar	38	76	12	24	0	0
3	P. Palya	26	52	24	48	0	0
4	A. Nagar	21	42	29	58	0	0
5	C. Nagar	0	0	23	58	27	54
	All Slums	99	39.6	124	49.6	27	10.8

Table-No. 46 - HIV/AIDS Awareness

Sl No	Name of the slum	Yes	Per centage	No	Per centage
1	B. Nagar	21	22	29	58
2	R. Nagar	41	82	9	18
3	P. Palya	37	74	13	26
4	A. Nagar	30	60	20	40
5	C. Nagar	30	60	20	40
All Slums		159	63.6	91	36.4

In spite of poor and limited knowledge about health and diseases on the one hand, it is surprising to note that 63.6 per cent of them are very much familiar about HIV/AIDS. This could be attributed to the severity of this disease, the importance given by the Government and non-governmental organisations in popularising the wild and ugly face of this disease and also may be because of the non-availability of treatment to it till today. On the other hand it is equally sad to note that in spite of all these efforts, there are a considerable *per cent* i.e., about 36.4 per cent who have replied to be unaware of this disease. From the preceding discussions, one can make an easy assessment of the knowledge attitude, perception and behaviours of slum dwellers regarding sex and related diseases.

Apart from this it is equally important to know about the perception attitude and behaviour of the slum dwellers with reference to Environment and related issues too.

Table-No. 47 - Does any of your family member have ever had this disease								
Sl No	Name of the slum	Yes	Per centage	No	Per centage	DK	Per centage	Total
1	B. Nagar	0	0	14	28	36	72	50
2	R. Nagar	0	0	36	72	14	28	50
3	P. Palya	0	0	26	52	24	48	50
4	A. Nagar	0	0	21	42	29	58	50
5	C. Nagar	0	0	22	14	28	86	50
All slums		0	0	119	47.6	131	52.4	250

It is strange to note that nobody has replied 'Yes' for the question asked about the occurrence of disease and this does not essentially mean that there is no such disease among the respondents or their family members instead it only reveals their views towards such diseases. About 47.6 per cent of the respondents have replied 'No' and this may be because of their ignorance about the disease or its existence or may be as discussed earlier lack of courage to disclose in view of getting bad name in the society.

Similarly, 52.4 per cent of them have replied to be unaware or ignorant about such issues which again highlight the need for bringing more awareness among them about the occurrence and symptoms of the disease so as to enable them to identify if so.

Table-No. 48 - Knowledge about precautions for safe sex:

Sl No	Name of the slum	Use of condom	per centage	Refuse to have sex with strangers (a)	per centage	Don't go to commercial sex workers (b)	per centage	(a) + (b) + (c)	per centage	D.K	per centage	No response	per centage	Total
1	B. Nagar	1	2	12	24	16	32	0	0	0	0	21	42	50
2	R. Nagar	6	12	1	2	14	28	7	14	17	34	5	10	50
3	P. Palya	25	50	2	4	1	2	8	16	4	8	10	20	50
4	A.Nagar	12	24	4	8	15	30	0	0	0	0	19	38	50
5	C. Nagar	7	14	7	14	16	32	0	0	0	0	20	40	50
	All slums	51	20.4	26	10.4	62	24.8	15	6	21	8.4	75	30	250

The table shows the level of knowledge and its implication in their regular course of life. 20.4 per cent of the sample has replied the use of condom is helpful for safe sex. 10.4 per cent has replied the refusal to have sex with strangers may be useful as another method for safe sex and 24.8 per cent have said the avoidance of contacts with commercial sex workers could also be of use in taking precautions about safe sex.

Table-No. 49 - What is the social and economic damage caused to the family by the habit of drinking

Sl No	Name of the slum	Economic instability	Per centage	Economic instability and Social abuse	Per centag	Economic instability, Social abuse, Physical abuse & bad effect on growing children	Per centag	Economic instability and bad effect on growing children	Per centag	Economic instability, Social abuse physical abuse	Per centag	No	Per centag	Do not know	Per centag	Total
1	B. Nagar	3	6	17	34	3	6	9	18	9	18	8	16	1	2	50
2	R. Nagar	28	56	1	2	10	20	8	16	0	0	0	0	0	0	50
3	P. Palya	15	30	0	0	10	20	2	4	5	10	5	10	23	46	50
4	A. Nagar	30	60	5	10	14	28	0	0	0	0	0	0	1	2	50
5	C. Nagar	21	42	5	10	13	26	5	10	4	8	0	0	2	4	50
All slums		97	38.8	28	11.2	50	20	24	9.6	18	7.2	13	5.2	27	10.8	250

Any person's behaviour irrespective of the situations has its impact on the family members in general and children in particular. This plays an important role in socialisation of the child. It tries to imitate the behaviour of the elders and follow it. Hence, it becomes very much necessary that the elderly members of the family should take care while enacting their roles. Here, 11.2 per cent of the respondents opine that the habit of drinking can cause economic instability along with social abuse while, 20 per cent of them is of the opinion that it can cause economic instability, social abuse, physical abuse and also bad effect on growing children. 9.6 per cent of them said that it has both economic implications and affect children's growth. 7.2 per cent of them feel that it may result in economic instability, social abuse and physical abuse while 5.2 per cent of them say that it can make no harm and cannot have any bad effect as such and 10.8 per cent of them seem to be unaware of the implications it can have on the family members. Here another striking point to be noted is that all of them accept that whether it may have or not have other implications but, economic implications are very much felt.

This question was posed with an intention to cull out information about the various kinds of trees and plants present in their surrounding environment and 13.2 per cent of them said that there are show plants near their residence most of them being personally planted. We can say that there is lack of Corporation initiative to provide green cover in these areas as only 3.6 per cent of corporation trees including Aralikattes are found. A negligible number i.e., 0.8 per cent of vegetable and fruit yielding plants are mentioned. Aralikattes seem to be the one and only green cover in these areas which amount to 17.2 per cent. More than half i.e., about 59.2 per cent sample has told to have no greenery in their surrounding environment. This being the situation in slums not to speak of city area as it has literally become the concrete jungle. This shows the pathetic

Table-No. 50 - Kind of trees present in the area

Sl No	Name of the slum	Show plant	Per centage	Corporation trees & arali katte	Per centage	Medicinal plant	Per centage	Vegetables and fruits	Per centage	Arali katte	Per centage	Any other	Per centage	No	Per centage	Total
1	B. Nagar	2	4	3	6	0	0	0	0	7	14	0	0	38	76	50
2	R. Nagar	0	0	0	0	1	2	0	0	17	34	0	0	32	64	50
3	P. Palya	6	12	0	0	8	16	0	0	0	0	0	0	36	72	50
4	A. Nagar	0	0	3	6	0	0	1	2	4	8	0	0	42	84	50
5	C. Nagar	25	50	3	6	12	24	1	2	6	12	3	6	0	0	50
	All slums	33	13.2	9	3.6	21	8.4	2	0.8	34	13.6	3	1.2	148	59.2	250

condition of the so called garden City of India. This is the emergency call of the hour to save the lives of ourselves and our future generation on this Mother Earth.

Table-No. 51 - What are the advantages you get from these plants?

Sl No	Name of the slum	Shadow	Per centage	Fresh air	Per centage	Shadow and fresh air	Per centage	Shadow, fresh air, fruits and vegetables	Per centage	Money/ Income	Per centage	Total
1	B. Nagar	2	4	2	4	40	80	6	12	0	0	50
2	R. Nagar	46	92	2	4	0	0	0	0	2	4	50
3	P. Palya	46	92	2	4	0	0	1	2	1	2	50
4	A. Nagar	32	64	4	8	8	16	1	2	5	10	50
5	C. Nagar	24	48	4	8	8	16	8	16	6	12	50
	All slums	**150**	**60**	**14**	**5.6**	**56**	**22.4**	**16**	**6.4**	**14**	**5.6**	**250**

The above table throws light on the knowledge of the slum residents on the usufructs of plants and trees. It can be seen that though they are residing in urban areas their rural background still finds a place in their attitudes and behaviour. Majority of them accept that they can get shadow (88.8 per cent) from the trees apart from getting fresh air (34.4 per cent), fruits and vegetables (6.4 per cent) and also some income (5.6 per cent) if possible.

Table-No. 52 – Details of pet animals

Sl No	Name of the slum	Cat	Per centage	Dog	Per centage	NO	Per centage	Total
1	B.Nagar	0	0	13	26	37	74	50
2	R.Nagar	7	14	7	14	36	72	50
3	P.Palya	2	4	8	16	40	80	50
4	A.Nagar	2	4	4	8	44	88	50
5	C.Nagar	1	2	11	22	38	76	50
All slums		12	4.8	43	17.2	195	78	250

From the time immemorial, man has been fond of animals and has always tried to rear, tame and nurture one or the other kind of animal irrespective of it being carnivorous or herbivorous. These animals have become his partners in all walks of life. In such a case, having pet animals is a habit found in human beings in general and it has also become the trend of the day in cities. To have a pet is a matter of prestige and fashion. But, slum dwellers struggling hard to find two meals a day can we expect them to have a pet and take care of it? In spite of this, 4.8 per cent of them are having cats and 17.2 per cent of them have dogs. The remaining 78 per cent of them do not possess any pets.

Table-No. 53 - How to check malnutrition

Sl No	Name of the slum	Nutritious food	Per centage	Personal hygiene & Nutritious food	Per centage	Not Applicable	Per centage	Total
1	B. Nagar	37	74	10	20	3	6	50
2	R. Nagar	49	98	1	2	0	0	50
3	P. Palya	49	98	0	0	1	2	50
4	A. Nagar	46	92	1	2	3	6	50
5	C. Nagar	49	98	0	0	1	2	50
All slums		230	92	12	4.8	8	3.2	250

Malnutrition is one of the common health problems faced by children in India. In India great number of children irrespective of poor or rich background suffers from malnutrition. The major reason attributed to this is the lack of knowledge about required intake of food by the children and certain blind beliefs avoiding them by feeding children with sufficient calories of food. Even personal hygiene also acts as a contributing factor for this. Majority of the respondents are aware that malnutrition can be supplemented with nutritious food but the problem lies in deciding what nutritious food is and how to administer it. 96.8 per cent of the respondents have replied that malnutrition could be controlled by providing nutritious food out of which 4.8 per cent feel that not only nutritious food but, personal hygiene should also be accompanied to get high results in this direction. Only a small per cent of about 3.2 per cent are unaware of this issue.

Table-No. 54 - Effect of domestic violence affect children's future

Sl No	Name of the slum	Yes	Per centage	No	Per centage	D.K	Per centage	Total
1	B. Nagar	20	40	26	52	4	8	50
2	R. Nagar	14	28	35	70	1	2	50
3	P. Palya	8	16	42	84	0	0	50
4	A. Nagar	12	24	38	76	0	0	50
5	C. Nagar	15	30	31	62	4	8	50
All slums		**69**	**27.6**	**172**	**68.8**	**9**	**3.6**	**250**

Domestic violence is a factor which essentially affects the growth of children. The child tries to imitate and follow elders in the process of socialisation. Hence, it is rightly said, 'home is the first school and mother is the first teacher'. When viewed with this background, one can rightly say that domestic violence do affect the growth particularly mental growth among children. Many studies conducted on the deviant and delinquent behaviour among children have revealed that the relationship among the members of the family and the living environment are major contributors. In spite of this many a times we neglect the influence of domestic violence on children. This is also evident from the table as only 27.6 per cent of the respondents are of the opinion that domestic violence may affect the growth of children. The major chunk of the group of about 68.8 per cent opines that it hardly has any effect on the growth of children. The remaining 3.6 per cent have reported to be unaware of this factor.

Table-No. 55 - Effect of domestic violence on neighbours

Sl No	Name of the slum	Yes	Per centage	No	Per centage	D.K	Per centage	Total
1	B. Nagar	3	6	45	90	2	4	50
2	R. Nagar	11	22	36	72	3	6	50
3	P. Palya	9	18	40	80	1	2	50
4	A. Nagar	8	16	40	80	2	4	50
5	C. Nagar	11	22	35	70	4	8	50
All slums		42	16.8	196	78.4	12	4.8	250

Though domestic violence appears to be purely personal and confined to a particular family it is not so. Apart from the members of the family, the neighbouring families also have to bear the heat of this problem. But unfortunately, the creators of this problem never understand this fact and if anybody tries to interfere and solve the problem the reply would be it is purely personal problem and no interference of outsiders would be entertained. Hence, 78.4 per cent of the respondents opine that the domestic violence hardly has anything to do with the neighbours and does not harm them. Only 16.8 per cent of them feel that it may affect the neighbours too. The remaining 4.8 per cent are not even aware of the problem as such.

Table-No. 56 - Effect of domestic violence on health								
Sl No	Name of the slum	Yes	Per centage	No	Per centage	D.K	Per centage	Total
1	B. Nagar	8	16	29	58	13	26	50
2	R. Nagar	11	22	4	8	35	70	50
3	P. Palya	10	20	30	60	10	20	50
4	A. Nagar	5	10	36	72	9	18	50
5	C. Nagar	10	20	9	18	31	62	50
All slums		**44**	**17.6**	**108**	**43.2**	**98**	**39.2**	**250**

Domestic violence leads to physical abuse and end up with man handling in most of the cases. This invariably affects the health of the subjugated both physical and mental. Not to speak of the by-products it may create out of it. In this table, 17.6 per cent of the respondents have replied that it has effect on health while, 43.2 per cent of them said it may not have any effect. 39.2 per cent of them are not even able to decide whether it may or may not have and hence, replied to be not aware of.

Table-No. 57 - Effect of domestic violence on society								
Sl No	Name of the slum	Yes	Per centage	No	Per centage	D.K	Per centage	Total
1	B. Nagar	1	2	26	52	23	46	50
2	R. Nagar	11	22	0	0	39	78	50
3	P. Palya	4	8	40	80	6	12	50
4	A. Nagar	2	4	40	80	8	16	50
5	C. Nagar	9	18	34	68	7	14	50
All slums		**27**	**10.8**	**140**	**56**	**83**	**33.2**	**250**

Given the above background, one can say that domestic violence also has its influence on the society as a whole. When questioned to our respondents, 10.8 per cent of them replied that it has effect on society whereas, 56 per cent of them said that it does not have any effect on society as it is personal and confined a particular family and about 33.2 per cent of them said that they cannot say anything on this.

Table-No. 58 - Have seen in your area these activities

Sl No	Name of the slum	Theft and Molestation	Per centage	Molestation	Per centage	Theft, Rape and Molestation	Per centage	Total
1	B. Nagar	19	38	28	56	3	6	50
2	R. Nagar	39	78	11	22	0	0	50
3	P. Palya	31	62	19	38	0	0	50
4	A. Nagar	7	14	43	86	0	0	50
5	C. Nagar	25	50	25	50	0	0	50
All slums		121	48.4	126	50.4	3	1.2	250

When questioned about various anti-social activities occurring in their living areas, the respondents have replied as follows: Molestation seems to be quite common and has often been seem happening in their vicinity and 48.4 per cent of the sample reported to have experienced theft. Rape is another thing often reported happening in the slums, though 1-2 per cent of the sample reported to have seen it happening.

Discussion of the analysis of empirical data has shown that human behaviour has much to do with environmental changes and the solution to environmental problems has got to be found in the dynamics of behavioural changes. Over population and population growth is one of the fundamental developments causing environmental problems (Ehrlich and Ehrlich, 1990, Shaw, 1992). Population growth is determined by the inter play of birth rate death rate and migration of people. A determined effort to limit the life span for the purpose of environmental preservation is not acceptable in today's society. On the other hand, every one is the more or less free to limit his or her reproduction voluntarily for environmental reasons.

The number of persons per household is decreasing in most countries, which also imply a larger number of households. The result is that on average all individuals are occupying more room and less space is available for functions other than dwellings. Firstly the tradition of different generations living together has decreased and secondly of couples living together has decreased. The increases in spacing are supporting growth in mobility as well. Motorised personal transport also contributes to many environmental problems (OECD, 1995). In many cases urban planning is limiting the possibilities for environmentally sound waves of traveling, like walking or cycling. Every person, to a certain degree, has a stable Behavioural patter in accordance with personal values, social norms and his or her personal living conditions. Concepts of environmental awareness and environmental concern were introduced, which are used for two purposes. The trends discussed in Behavioural patterns are responsible for increased environmental problems, because consumption growth is causing an increase in the use environmental functions. The decision for public transport is a positive one compared with driving a car but it is negative compared with cycling.

One way or another within all our daily behaviour there are hardly any actions that do not result in some environmental stress. Behaviour that is partially motivation by the consequences of the acts for the environment is mostly categorised as 'ecologically sound' or 'environmentally sound'. Looking at above figure it is obvious that these terms are not as unambiguous as they are often presented. In the hole range of behaviour with a certain relevance to the environment five types may be distinguished. For this typology to criteria are used: the physical effect of the behaviour (whether or not it affects the environment) and the social meaning of the behaviour (negative versus positive).

Sociologists and Social anthropologists define certain patterns of behaviour which influence environment both negatively and positively. Environmental management strategies have got to be design with a view to curbing and discouraging if necessary punishing human behaviour which might be actually harmful to environment. For example, Supreme Court orders in banning smoking in public place. Human behaviour which contributes to environmental protection must be encouraged by means of environmental education.

This is a category of behaviour with environmental consequences that are easy to avoid. The impact may easily be reduced by choosing alternative that are more environmentally sound.

This is the category of behaviour consisting of alternatives for type I behaviour. Three are two possibilities. First: behaviour that is causing environmental treble that replaces behaviour with severe environmental consequences. For example: going to work by public transport instead of a car. Second: operations that are limiting environmental impact that are an extension of existing behaviour. If a clear choose is made for these alternatives for reasons linked to the avoidance of environmental impact, behaviour of this type may be called 'environmentally sound'. An example is separating house hold waste, which is not limiting the amount of waste but creating an opportunity to reduce land fill and incineration.

This is the largest category, but also invisible in most cases because it includes acts with environmental impact that are not conducted. This is the most important environmentally sound category of behaviour. Nevertheless it is hardly recognised because there is a whole range of motives for it and many of these motives are not linked to any kind of ecological consideration. With in this category a distinction should be made between type 3a, environmentally motivated behaviour, and type 3b, with out environmental motives.

Any kind of behaviour conducted for recovery of environmental damage or the prevention of it belongs to this category. Examples are participation in environmental actions or the support of environmental organisation or participation in pollution prevention activities such as reuse of products or the use of recycled products. A more direct type which is in most cases institutional behaviour, is cleaning polluted soil, planting trees, recovering damaged ecosystems by re-introducing species. This fourth behaviour is easily recognised as environmentally sound as the motives are predominantly ecological.

This is a category of mostly institutional behaviour without direct environmental impact. It is directed at maintaining or extending the possibilities for environmentally unsound behavioural alternatives. The way many products are offered in package which consumers often consider oversised and unnecessary, is an example. Another striking example is the installation in buildings of appliances which cannot be switched off, for instance lighting, ventilation, air-conditioners or automatic awnings.

Empirical research on behaviour which is relevant for the environment mostly shows hardly any correlation between concrete types of behaviour. The reason is that there are no social or psychological criteria primarily determining whether or not behaviour is relevant to the environment. The criteria for characterisation of behaviour are of a physical nature, lying beyond social or psychological categories. Because there is no common human origin, behaviour relevant for the environment cannot be described within one dimension. There are no common origins, only common results (environmental damage) and in general these results are only side effects of human behaviour.

Data on public perception of the environmental issues are interesting as an indicator of the attention paid to the environment with in society public opinion time series-data show changing attention and concern, cross-sectional research may indicate significant variation between countries are population group. How can these variation be explained and can they be interpreted in terms of growing significance of new environmental values? What is environmental awareness? Is there actually an increasing significance of it? And is this awareness founded in changing values?

Table-No. 59 – Reason for death

Sl No	Name of the slum	TB	Per centage	Heavy drinks	Per centage	Aged	Per centage	Paralysis (Stroke)	Per centage	Heart attack	Per centage
1	B. Nagar	1	2	0	0	4	8	0	0	0	0
2	R. Nagar	3	6	1	2	1	2	0	0	0	0
3	P. Palya	3	6	0	0	1	2	0	0	0	0
4	A. Nagar	0	0	1	2	1	2	0	0	1	2
5	C. Nagar	2	4	0	0	0	0	1	2	0	0
All slums		9	3.6	2	0.8	7	2.8	1	0.4	1	0.4

The above tries to give the details of reasons for death occurred in slums. Tuberculosis appears to be one of the prominent reasons for death among the elderly people, 3.6 per cent the highest among the given reasons being this. This disease though prevalent among slum dwellers, the number deaths due to this are minimised presently because of the efforts made by the Government and NGOs in persuading them to undergo the DOT (Direct Observation Therapy) treatment. The intensive efforts put in by these sectors in bringing awareness among them and the belief of getting cured has made the programme successful to a greater extent. 2.8 per cent being the age factor responsible for the death, which is the most unavoidable and natural reason causing death. 0.8 per cent has said to be died because of heavy drinking being one of the major social problems in our society. Only a small *per cent* of about 0.4 per cent has died due to paralysis and heart attack. This may be because of the food habits among the slum residents i.e., when having two meals a day being hard earned the possibilities of getting heart attacks due to excess cholesterol in the body becomes unimaginable. The junk and oily food habits among the high society people have made them more vulnerable to these kinds of diseases, the polluted environment being one of the important factors in increasing the health risks of the city residents in general and slum residents in particular.

CHAPTER VI
ENVIRONMENTAL MOVEMENTS

Environmental movments and role of NGOs in environmental Movements

Widely called 'new social movements', Environmental Movements are so called because they don't subscribe atleast explicitly to any class ideologies and that they are committed to holistic approach to development and that local communities must enjoy the fruits of development. Environmental movements have been the most dramatic and visible social movements in the post-World War period. "Earth Day 1970, is often said to represent the debut of the modern environmental movement" (Hannigan 1997; 5). Concern with interaction between physical environment and social organisation and behaviour is as old as sociology. Lack of common theoretical thread in sociological studies of environment has been recognised though rather belatedly. Existing literature on environmental sociology has related rather overwhelmingly with, a) The causes of environmental destruction, b) The rise of environmental consciousness and movements. Reason for dramatic rise in the environmental movements and environmental consciousness have been discussed very lucidly (*Ibid*, 23, 31). The fact of the matter, however is that nothing whatsoever ever becomes an issue much less an environmental issue unless people concerned perceive, define and articulate it as an issue. The phenomena of environmental issues have a great deal to do with dynamics of human behaviour. The role of social activist groups occupies an important and significant place in the preservation, conservation and protection of environment and environmental management.

What then is an environmental movement? "One may define an environmental movement as organised social activity directed towards promoting sustainable use of natural resources, halting environmental degradation or bringing about environmental restoration." Modern environmental movements had helped to make sociologists more aware of the human-nature interaction.

Mukerjee emphasises that the relationship between nature and nurture and culture is both interactive dynamic, with human trying to mould environment to their own ends but always having to work with in the limited set by nature (Guha; 1998-19, 20).

Unabated proliferation of voluntary action group over the last two decades has marked the beginning of environmental movements in India. The Chipko movement in earstwhile Uttar Pradesh Himalayas, which has played a vital role in bringing the issues of deforestation to the fore front of public opinion, the Appiko movement in the Western Ghats of Karnataka has been major force to reckon with, which has brought about environmental consciousness among the people at the grass root level. Dams like Silent Valley and Bedthi have already been stopped because of people's strong protest. There has been a major campaign against the proposed Bhopalapatnam and Inchampally dams on the borders of the Madhya Pradesh, Andhra Pradesh and Maharastra.

Kerala Sastra Sahitya Parishad (KSSP) has had protracted battle over the pollution of Chaliyar River by rayon mill. The India Development Service finds itself caught in controversy over river pollution by Rayon Mill in Karnataka. The Shadhol Group has been waging a heroic battle against the pollution of a river in Shadhol district by a paper mill. The Mitti Bachao Abhiyan has been organising farmers against water logging caused by faulty irrigation system.

Needless to add most of these groups have been doing excellent work in mobilising and organising people at the local grass root level. They have been getting good co-operation and support from the media both print as well as electronic not speak of strong support ungrudgingly extended by what has come to be known as Judicial activism (See the previous chapter), intellectuals and environmentally sensitive human rights activist groups. For, conflicts over the preservation, use and control of natural resources almost inevitably often boils down to inter-caste and inter-class conflicts. Environmental degradation in India has almost always followed the misuse and abuse of natural resources by vested interest. The main agenda of the environmental movements, among much else, is basically three folds- 1) to prevent further ecological destruction. 2) Bring about ecological regeneration. 3) To put environment at the service and control of the people, the people usually being defined as the local communities who live within that environment. (Agarwal, 1998, 347-348).

ENVIRONMENT SUPPORT GROUP ®

The Organisation:

Environment Support Group (ESG) is an independent not-for-profit non-governmental organisation, registered as a Trust. Its main functions involve research, training, campaign, support, and advocacy on a variety of environmental and social justice issues. Environment Support Group started in 1996 informally as Bangalore Support Group. Following its informal association with various NGOs and Campaigns as a consultant, it was established as an independent non-profit Trust in April 1998.

ESG has worked with a wide range of organisations and coalitions at the local, regional, national and international levels in a variety of collaborations. An illustrative list includes: At the International level: United Nations Environment Programme, United Nations Economic and Social Commission for Asia and the Pacific, Asia Urban Programme of the European Commission, Environment Law Institute, One World, Export Credit Agencies Reform Campaign, The Tides Foundation/Green Grants, Friends of the Earth-Japan, Association for India's Development, International Honors Program/Boston University, SANA-South Asia North America Environmental Justice

The Initiative

At the National level: Involving and supporting campaigns of various coalitions and associations against environmental destruction and social injustice including Environmental Justice Initiative, Conservation and Livelihoods Network, the Right to Information network, and various Ministries of the Government. At the regional level: With National Law School of India University, Bangalore, Karnataka Dept. of Ecology and Environment, Indo-Norwegian Environment Programme and various local governments.

At the local community level: Supporting Public Campaigns and Public Interest Litigations of Janajagriti Samithi of Nandikur (Udupi Dt.), Vimana Nildhana Vistharana Virodhi Samithi of Bajpe (Mangalore), Save Kudremukh from Mining Campaign (Chickamagalur Dt.), Parisara Samrakshana Samithi (Sirsi), Save Cubbon Park Campaign (Bangalore), Save Arkavathy Campaign (Bangalore), Shambavi River Protection Committee (Karkala), amongst others.

The main functions of ESG are in the following areas

Research functions include a range of activities from broad-based research initiatives such as monitoring and identifying major policy and investment decisions and their impacts, to conducting specific research into individual projects to understand their socio-economic and environmental impacts. We continuously update such information and feed-forward to a various civil society organisations in order to influence various decision making levels of the Government.

Documentation and Publication involves specific focus on issues of law and policy relating to Environment and Conservation. We monitor developments, investments and policies by sourcing of a variety of literature (newspaper and magazines, scientific journals, company profiles, government orders, policy statements, etc.) and make it available to campaigns, training initiatives, media advocacy, lobbying, public interest litigation's (PILs), publications, etc. Legal Support to local communities and campaign networks to access various legally mandated avenues in ensuring social and environmental justice concerns are not compromised in decisions affecting their life and livelihood. When need arises this relationship advances to supporting Public Interest Litigation by enabling the affected communities to represent their cause by litigation documentation and providing public interest lawyering support. ESG has independently initiated or intervened with PILs on certain issues when needed. Training involves development of training modules and conducting of workshops on a range of topics such as environment and social justice issues, legislation and policies, perspectives of development, alternatives, campaign strategies, etc. for a variety of focus groups at local and regional levels. Campaign activities involve addressing issues of environmental and social justice concern with local communities, the media, administration, legislature, judiciary, business community, etc.

Activities of ESG:

Projects

Community Access 2000: ESG has successfully facilitated a bid for Raichur Municipal Council of Karnataka under the new initiative of European Commission - Asia Urbs. Amongst a select few cities selected across Asia, the project, COMMUNITY ACCESS 2000, will be implemented over two years in partnership with London Borough of Brent, and Horsens and Health International of Denmark. ESG would be involved in its capacity as Associate Partner and Programme Coordinator on behalf of Raichur in the delivery of the project involving a comprehensive effort to improve urban, environmental, social and health planning for the city of Raichur located in the backward North Karnataka region. In anticipation of the main project implementation, ESG has secured a small grant from National Foundation for India and German Technical Cooperation towards conducting a preliminary study of the Urbanisation processes in Raichur. In May 2002 a consultation workshop was facilitated by ESG in Raichur. The workshop was well attended by key local government leaders and community representatives thus presenting a unique forum where the community could interact with its elected representatives. Participants enthusiastically voiced their concerns about major social, economic and environmental issues in Raichur thus achieving one of the major aims of the workshop. This formed the output of the workshop and the basis on which further research and planning work would be undertaken. (2001 - ongoing) ESG has represented Raichur in a variety of national and international forums to present the effort including in the conference on "Cities, Poverty and Environment" organised by Hanoi People's Committee and City net at Hanoi, Vietnam (July 2001), "Cities of the Future" organised by Indian Ministry of Urban Affairs and European Union in Vigyan Bhavan, Delhi (October 2000) and "City Networking for a Sustainable Future and Human Unity" organised by Auroville (February 2002).

Alamatti Dam:

The contentious issue of raising the height of the Alamatti dam to 524 metres took another turn on April 23, 1999 with the Supreme Court of India directing Andhra Pradesh, Maharashtra, and the Union government to file responses to Karnataka's plea for interim orders on its proposals. Karnataka's proposal includes impounding water at RL 515.2 metres and annual utilisation at 155 tmc under the Upper Krishna Project, even after it completed the erection of all 26-crest gates to their full height of RL 524.256 metres, but without raising the existing solid crest level beyond 509 metres. The contention of Maharashtra is that at a height of 524 metres, the Alamatti dam would submerge substantial areas within that state. Andhra Pradesh too has filed a suit to prevent Karnataka from raising the dam's level, and has asked for relief in conformity with the Bachawat award that deals with the distribution and allocation of the Krishna waters. (Chetan Nagendra V Year, NLSIU Kadam B.E.)

Chiguru:

Chiguru meaning "to sprout" in Kannada is an innovative programme on environment and development issues in the context of Bangalore. Aimed at higher secondary and college students the programme seeks to use interactive techniques and experiential learning to promote an organic interest in the student of environment and development issues and the role they play in these processes. The learning revolves around 5 themes, each essential to life on earth: Agni (Fire), Jala (Water), Vayu (Wind), Prithvi (Earth), Akash (Ether) And Pran (Life). ESG is currently seeking funding for the programme that will cover 4 schools in one academic year. (June 2002, ongoing) Research Studies for UNESCAP: ESG conducted a year-long research exercise for the United Nations Economic and Social Commission for Asia and the Pacific on "Integrating Environmental Considerations in Economic Policy Decision Making - A Case Study of Dakshina Kannada." This study reviewed major industrial and infrastructural developments in the environmentally and culturally unique coastal (undivided) Dakshina Kannada district of Karnataka, especially in the context of the "globalisation" processes. A significant result of this study has been the review of the strengths and weaknesses of environmental decision making in India.

Consultant to National Law School:

ESG is consultant to the National Law School of India University (NLSIU), Bangalore in a variety of training and research initiatives. During 1998, ESG conducted a study for NLSIU and the Dutch agency NOVIB on "Evaluating the Implementation of the Right to Environment in Karnataka."

Research and Programme Initiatives:

Review of Environmental Decision-Making Cycles in India: On the suggestion of the Union Environment Minister, ESG volunteered a paper reviewing the functioning of the Ministry of Environment and Forests during October 2000 for the Regional Offices Meeting. The specific focus of this paper was the Environmental Decision Making cycles in India, and their inconsistencies with the growing need for transparency, public involvement and technical competence in project impact review. As a follow up to this initiative, ESG proposes to prepare a series of modules for training on environmental decision making steps so as to enable a campaign for reform of the laws, policies and guidelines in collaboration with NGOs, academics and regulatory agencies.

A "Manual/Training Package on the conduct of and participation in Statutory Environmental Public Hearings" is proposed for development by ESG in collaboration with

Karnataka State Dept of Environment. ESG is presently sourcing funding support for the project. International NGO Campaign to reform Export Credit Agencies: ESG is involved in the international effort to reform export credit agencies (ECAs) and ensure compliance with various human rights and environmental standards. ESG is preparing a database on Indian investments covered by various ECAs and plans to disseminate this information to build awareness about such processes. ESG was represented in the NGO Strategy Session held in Jakarta during May 2000.

Environmental Decision Making Processes in India:

A study of the Environmental Decision Making Processes in India, focusing on the need to limit the damage to environment and reduce conflict by integrating participatory processes in the decision making cycle and evolve a rationale for ecologically sensitive industrial and infrastructure development is a major focus of ESG's ongoing research. As part of this initiative, ESG has produced a recommendatory document proposing areas of reform in the functioning of the Ministry of Environment and Forests, at the behest of the Union Environment Minister, during October 2000.

Campaigns and Public Interest Litigations

Bangalore Mysore Infrastructure Corridor: ESG has been involved along with various citizens and community groups in the cities of Bangalore, Mysore, and Mandya in demanding access to environmental, techno-economic and social impact information on the Rs. 4,000 crores (Rs. 40 billion) Bangalore-Mysore Infrastructure Corridor proposed by M/s. Nandi Infrastructure Corridor Enterprise Ltd. The project involves potential dislocation (by certain estimates) of over 200,000 people and acquisition of over about 21,000 acres of land consisting of private farm-lands, wetlands and forests. In statutory Environmental Public Hearings on the project held during March 2000, ESG was instrumental in securing a commitment for divulging project information. Subsequently, the Government reneged on its commitment, proceeding to hold Adjourned Public Hearings during June and July, 2000. Citizens groups actively resisted this in Mysore, Mandya, and Bangalore, but the State responded with brutal police action selectively targeting individuals and groups pressing for transparency on the project.

A campaign condemning such action was initiated by ESG and received international support with the Chief Minister being pressurised for corrective action. ESG moved the National Human Rights Commission for an enquiry into human rights abuse and the Commission is enquiring into the petition. ESG exposed a major fraud in the project where the developers claimed the involvement of a US firm in the consortium, while that firm denies involvement in BMIC. These and other substantive details formed the basis of ESG's representation to the Ministry of Environment and Forests during May 2001. Despite acknowledging the validity of the representation, the Ministry extended a conditional environmental clearance to the project during August 2001. Efforts are on to challenge the validity of this decision. More recently, based on a representation made by ESG, the Reserve Bank of India (RBI) has filed a case against ICICI, a major financier of the project. ICICI may be violating a binding directive issued by the RBI in February 2002 regarding 'Financing of Infrastructure Projects' which warns against project financing based on state guarantees or comfort letters, as is the case in BMIC.

Campaign against the Cogentrix Power Project: ESG worked with Janajagriti Samithi (Public Awareness Committee) of Nandikur, in Dakshina Kannada, a committee of project affected communities, in sustaining their decade long resistance to the location of Thermal Power Plants in the environmentally sensitive and coastal Dakshina Kannada region.

Following the liberalisation of the Indian Economy, the power sector was provided special place for Foreign Direct Investment and the Mangalore Power Company, initially promoted by Cogentrix Inc. of USA, was selected as one of 8 "fast track" projects by the Indian Government, by facilitating speedy clearances in demonstrating its commitment to the liberalisation agenda. Human rights, environmental protection, sound economics and transparency in decision making were compromised in the process. The political apparatus played a significant role this travesty of governance. Here, ESG worked with the local project affected community to claim their rights and expose the serious ills in the project. This involved complete involvement and support in the Campaign and Public Interest Litigation against the project promoters, Cogentrix Inc. and China Light and Power (CLP), both in the High Court of Karnataka and Supreme Court of India. The litigation was initiated by Janajagriti Samithi and supported by then Member of Parliament, Ms. Maneka Gandhi (presently Union Minister of State for Social Justice and Empowerment). These petitions were filed on grounds of violations of environmental, social justice and planning norms. ESG deposed before the Supreme Court appointed NEERI commission enquiring into the environmental and social impact compliance of the project on behalf of Janajagriti Samithi. Consequently, the High Court of Karnataka called for a review of the project by Ministry of Environment.

A parallel initiative exposing the corruption in the project was initiated by Mr. Arun Kumar Agarwal, a finance consultant, and ESG facilitated his PIL initiative. The High Court of Karnataka convinced with the petitioners charges ordered an high level enquiry by the Central Bureau of Investigation into the project, but this ruling was subsequently stayed and dismissed by the Supreme Court. ESG also worked with the Jenks Neighbourhood Alliance Council of Jenks City, Oklahoma, and the local communities of Mississippi in their fight against Cogentrix investments that once more reflected lax implementation of accepted environmental and social standards. ESG facilitated a solidarity alliance between the affected communities, which significantly weakened the brazen approach Cogentrix had adopted in pushing its investment plans ahead disregarding accepted standards.

A combination of all these efforts resulted in Cogentrix and CLP announcing its withdrawal from the project on December 9th, 1999. Within days the Supreme Court delivered its controversial judgement exonerating the investors of corruption, following reservation of the order for almost a year. Subsequently, ESG has been involved in campaigning for a reopening of the case on the admittance by a Member of Legislative Assembly of Karnataka that he had been offered a large sum of money by Cogentrix in return for silence on the project's adverse implications. The pullout by Cogentrix consequent to this 7 year long campaign precipitated a situation wherein the Government of Karnataka was forced to set up a high level committee headed by Deepak Parekh to review the health of the State Energy Sector in supporting the various Independent Power Producers investments under escrow cover. The Committee rejected escrow cover for any investment given the poor financial health of the State Electricity Board, which resulted in the rejection of over 25 Power Purchase Agreements (PPAs) that had been negotiated through the highly controversial MOU route. The Karnataka Government accepted this report, and in turn influenced a National Policy to not accord any escrow cover to private investors.

In a furtive attempt, CLP resumed its involvement in the Mangalore Power Company in joint venture with Tata Electric of India. ESG and Janajagriti Samithi continue to challenge this project, and it appears that the project may be abandoned, thus weakening the possibility of Nagarjuna

Power Company to locate another 1,000 MW project in the same region as well. During March 2000, ESG was invited to present its case against Cogentrix in the Permanent People's Tribunal organised by the School of Law, University of Warwick, UK.

Dandeli Dam

ESG along with Parisara Samrakshana Kendra, Sirsi, ran a campaign to stop a dam proposed across the Kali River by the Murdeshwar Power Corporation Ltd. (MPCL). ESG exposed Ernst and Young, the international consulting firm, for plagiarising a Rapid Environment Impact Assessment (REIA) of Tattihalla Augmentation Scheme in preparing the REIA of the Dandeli dam in an attempt to secure clearances. In what was termed as the worst ever scam in environmental decision making history of India, Indian Express provided front page main coverage to the issue in all their country-wide editions on 27 August 2000, leading to a series of further stories across the world. Forced by such circumstances, the Karnataka Government ordered a fresh EIA for the project.

Despite all the controversy, Tata Energy Research Institute (TERI) which was commissioned to conduct this study produced the EIA within a month. On review this was found to be based on fraudulent data. In a Public Hearing held on the basis of this report on 3rd January 2001, the deposition made by ESG was considered substantive evidence against the TERI report, and the same was requested to be filed on affidavit by the District Commissioner of Uttara Kannada district. This file can be accessed along with selections from the plagiarised Ernst and Young report, considering the stance of the Karnataka Forest Department against allowing the dam construction, the project is likely to be abandoned. (2000-2001)

Save Arkavathi, Save Bangalore

In commemoration of the 1999 International Day of Action for Rivers, Water and Life of the International Rivers Network ESG facilitated a citizen's campaign against the decision of the Government of Karnataka to allow a massive luxury housing and recreation project of DLF Constructions in the watershed of River Arkavathi, providing about a third of Bangalore's water supply. Sanmathi women's group led this campaign in which with over 200 citizens groups and pressurised the Chief Minister of Karnataka to declare the area ecologically sensitive. Recently, the Government has proposed to declare an area of 10 kms radius of the Rivers watershed as no-development zone for all industrial and urban developments.

a) Save Cubbon Park Campaign:

ESG helped initiate the sensational Save Cubbon Park Campaign during September 1998 in collaboration with Sanmathi women's group, fighting against encroachment aided by the Legislators and the Government of one of Bangalore's landmark and historic park spaces. The issue that started with ESG calling for people's involvement snowballed into a major movement that saw daily rallies by thousands involving students, community organisations, professional organisations, etc. for over a month. Due to such wide public pressure the High Court was compelled to stay the Government order to de-notify a major portion of the Park and divert it for building.

This resulted in a controversy, bringing the Legislature in loggerheads with the Judiciary for intervening to stay the Government's order. The Judiciary whilst staying the operation of the Government notification had also called for a ban on protests against the Government action and this resulted in a civil rights debate in the National Press with human rights activist Justice H. Suresh criticising the Court for curtailing civil rights as well. ESG enabled a symbolic protest against this "ban" as a threat against the Right to Express, even as it impleaded into the ongoing litigation to protect the Park permanently. The High Court has dismissed this petition during August 2001 and ESG proposes to appeal this decision in the Supreme Court.

This campaign was supported by leading theatre personalities including Jnanpith awardee Mr. Girish Karnad, Ms. Medha Patkar of the Narmada Bachao Andolan, Justice H. Suresh, Justice Nittoor Srinivasa Rao and artists, writers, students, academicians, community based groups, etc. The Save Cubbon Park Campaign was widely reported across the country and inspired a wave of protests and alliances against the encroachment of public spaces by predatory businesses, politicians and communal forces.

b) The Tragedy of Bellandur

Bangalore has an extremely well planned lake system. These lakes formed the lifeline of the residents of various localities in the city. Over the years, most of the lakes have been subjects of neglect and misuse. As a result, there are many that have gone dry. The remaining ones are polluted unimaginably. The Bellandur Lake belongs to the latter category. CEERA's association with the Bellandur lake issue began with a visit to the lake at the request of Dr.Yellappa Reddy, the well-known conservationist. Members of the CEERA team participated in a consultative meeting with the local people and the Panchayat officials. In the course of the meeting, certain startling facts were brought to light.

The Bellandur Lake is a few kilometres from the Bangalore Airport. The lake is huge - about 950 acres. The major *per cent*age of the sewage generated by Bangalore city is being let into the lake in an untreated form. In fact, the lake is found to contain pollutants a staggering 160 times more than permissible levels. Despite repeated requests, the authorities had been unwilling to act and the matter had been taken to the High Court of Karnataka. The local population is suffering a variety of privations as a result of the polluted lake and they sought legal advice to have their problems alleviated. The members of the CEERA team gave their suggestions as to the possible legal avenues open to the Panchayat. It was decided at the consultative meeting that a multi-pronged strategy, using all the available legal tools should be employed. Awareness about the lake's plight had to be generated among the city-dwellers.

To this end, a press meet was organised and press-persons were invited to visit the lake. The result was widespread coverage of the issue in the media. At the same time, the High Court took serious note of the matter and issued notice to the authorities concerned to explain the action taken so far as regards the retrieval of the lake. Further developments are awaited and hopefully, one of the largest of Bangalore's lakes will be on the road to recovery.

For the CEERA team, it was a chance to see law-in-action and in that sense, a learning experience. The members of the team were encouraged by the fact that their suggestions were met with great enthusiasm. (Input taken from, S.A. Karthik)

c) Media View Point: Green Issues

Thippa Gondana Halli

The media has been playing a vital role in following up environmental issues and bringing it to the knowledge of the public at large. The Cubbon Park issue is one such outstanding example. It brought to the general public the problem that the most vital lung space in Bangalore faced, until the matter became subjudice. Similarly, another important role that the media played was with respect to the case of the T.G. Halli reservoir.

The T.G. Halli issue involved the conversion of certain agricultural lands to non-agricultural lands in order to build some flats. The proposed construction was to have come up close to the T.G. Halli reservoir, one of the major water supply sources to the city. It was apprehended the source, would be polluted and blocked as a result of the development activities. The government however proposed to approve the conversion. And here, the vital role of the media, especially newspapers has to be highlighted. Through a close scrutiny of the developments in the case, public opinion was gradually built and perhaps, not since the Cubbon Park issue was public participation in an environmental issue so prominent. What it essentially achieved was, to make people aware of environmental problem, and the legal arguments that arise in environmental related matters. The conflicts in the administrative structure were also clearly brought out in the various reports. Public opinion began to mount, largely against the project. Finally, the government withdrew the permission, though the Supreme Court of India had ruled in favour of the project. The decision was unprecedented. Never had a government that had a favourable ruling withdrawn its earlier decision.

People's movement across the country claimed a substantial victory with the Karnataka Government's decision not to go ahead with the TG Halli Township. The Thippagondanahalli Reservoir is one of the primary sources of water to the city of Bangalore. The State Government had given permission to a Delhi based company to construct 270 villas in the catchment area of the reservoir. The Karnataka HC had quashed the clearance to the Project, but the SC revoked the order in an appeal. Interestingly, the Bangalore Water Supply and Sewerage Board (BWSSB) has been foremost in the opposition to the project stating that it could cause serious pollution to the vital water source. This clearly shows that public participation and opinion in shaping the law matter.

ESG-One world Website Development Training for NGOs:

A 4 day "Website Development Training Workshop" was organised by ESG in collaboration with One World - South Asia at the software training centre of SASKEN Communication Technologies Ltd., the sponsor, from18-21st January 2001. Over 15 NGOs and people's organisations participated in the workshop, and achieved the purpose of setting up the trial websites. This was the second such initiative of ESG with One World - South Asia, the first being a similar training conducted 30th October – 1st November 1999 in collaboration with One World (South Asia) and sponsored by Philips Software at its Software Development Centre. Over 20 NGOs from Karnataka and Tamil Nadu had benefited then. Post-workshop training is enabled by way of email discussion groups and by holding refresher courses. The effort is to help build Web Solidarity amongst NGOs and direct stories on a variety of environment, development and human rights initiative onto the One World website. (Report is available.) A 3 day residential experiential workshop on the "Environmental and Developmental Challenges of Bangalore" was organised by ESG in collaboration with the Rotary Club of Bangalore (South Parade), 30thJuly to 1stAugust, 1999. Participants included media persons, NGO, CBO and Government representatives and activists. Learning experiences were organised by field exposure to a variety of issues including urban planning, pollution and waste management, traffic management, slum living conditions, environmental health, judicial interventions, energy demands and power sector planning, biological control of urban weed problems, etc. The programme secured the active involvement of experts from the Bangalore Water Supply and Sewerage Board, Karnataka State Forest Department, Karnataka State Police Department (Traffic Cell), Biological Control Research Laboratories, Karnataka Dept. of Forest, Ecology and Environment, etc.

ESG conducted a Workshop on the "The Truth about the Cogentrix Deal" during June 1997 in collaboration with the National Alliance of People's Movement and Janajagriti Samithi. This was attended by leading media representatives and public interest advocates. Leading expert discussants included energy experts Dr. Amulya K. N. Reddy of the International Energy Initiative, Dr. V. Ranganathan of the Indian Institute of Management, and Dr. D. K. Subramanian of the Indian Institute of Science.

Mulki Under Seige: A training/campaign workshop was held by ESG at Padubidri, Dakshina Kannada in collaboration with Janajagriti Samithi, Nandikur, and with support from the National Environmental Awareness Campaign of the Ministry of Environment and Forests. The workshop participants, being local villagers, academicians, lawyers and the media, involved in making a mass representation to the Union Environment Minister Suresh Prabhu to not allow the proposed location of the Cogentrix and Nagarjuna thermal power stations on the banks of the ecologically fragile Mulki estuary and take action against the Engelhard Corporation for illegally developing a pigment facility at the source of the river. ESG periodically supports experiential training programmes for student groups. Some work in this area include advising the Law Reform Project of the National Law School of India University, supporting Global Ecology Programme of the International Honours Programme, Rotary Foundation, Centre for Environment Education, Student Projects of Indian Institute of Management-Bangalore, Institute of Finance and International Management-Bangalore and various local schools and colleges.

Media Campaign

As part of its advocacy work ESG has conducted/ supported over 50 Press conferences on a variety of public interest issues in collaboration with its partners.

International Honors Programme

ESG in collaboration with Arunodaya Poirada (NGO) organizes a month long Study Abroad experiential educational programme entitled "Cities of the 21st Century" of the International Honours Programme, an accredited academic course with the Bard College and Boston University, USA. Over 30 students drawn from Universities across the USA and 4 Travelling Faculty are facilitated by ESG in their study of ecological, cultural and economic dynamics of Chennai, Bangalore, Mysore and Raichur cities in India. The exposure includes stay in villages affected by the Bangalore Mysore Infrastructure Corridor project. ESG has facilitated this programme during 2003 and 2003 and it appears that this would be a regular feature of ESG-IHP collaboration. (January-February 2003, 2002). Solid Waste Management Training Initiative: In collaboration with the Human Health and Well Being Division of United Nations Environment Programme ESG initiated a pilot project aimed at developing the capacities of Pourakarmikas (municipal solid waste workers) of one Health Ward of the Bangalore Mahanagara Palike in evolving a sustainable strategy for management of community level municipal solid waste. As part of this project an evaluation of the work conditions of Pourakarmikas was undertaken with the aim of proposing suitable changes in appropriately managing this crucial workforce of the city. The scope of the project has now expanded with the support of the Karnataka Dept. of Environment under the Indo-Norwegian Environment Programme, and is likely to be the basis of intervention in Bangalore and other cities as well. Products of this project include a flipchart explaining the need for and instructions on separation of waste, and Nagara Nyrmalya an entertaining and informative short film which explores the complex issues of the community's role in solid waste management, and how Santhimmi, a Pourakarmika, motivates people in her neighbourhood to adopt safe solid waste management techniques. Due to the success of the programme, INEP has asked ESG to expand this programme in six more cities of Karnataka.

CENTRE FOR ENVIRONMENTAL LAW, EDUCATION, RESEARCH AND ADVOCACY (CEERA)

CEERA, NLSIU is planning to come out with a journal on Environmental Law by October 1999. The theme of the journal, the first of its kind in India, is 'Environmental Law in India'. Contributions for the same can be made, either in the form of articles, notes and book or case reviews. The same must reach CEERA by 10th September 1999. The contributions must be typed and if possible, the same be sent by e-mail and in floppy. (Bibhu Prasad Tripathy-CEERA)

With the object of consolidating the existing efforts on and pay focused attention to the ever evolving frontier area of environmental law, CEERA was brought into existence in the academic year 1997-98. This Centre for Excellence in Environmental Law signifies the second phase of evolution of the NLSIU.

- Teaching and Research
- Training and Advocacy
- Publications
- Environmental Law Consultancy Services in CEERA
- Projects
- Case Studies
- About CEERA Team

Teaching and Research:

Teaching has acquired a new meaning at CEERA. Being interactive and inter disciplinary in nature, the teaching here offers abundant scope for participatory learning. A foundation course in environmental law; optional seminar courses in Natural Resources and Energy Law and

International Environmental Law and an optional clinical course in Environmental Advocacy, for the the students of B.A. LL.B. (Hons) is offered. At the Post-Graduate level specialisation in Environmental Law is offered to students. A course in Environmental Law has been specially designed for the students of the Distance Education programme in Master of Business Laws. In order to meet the increasing demand for Environmental Law education, CEERA also offers a One Year Post-Graduate Diploma in Environmental Law. A number of doctoral research works are being carried out at the centre as also field-oriented research work, in different parts of India.

Training and Advocacy

As an on going process, teaching, training and capacity building in Environmental Law, is being offered to, the managers of environment in India. Government Functionaries, Industrial Managers, Judges, Law Practitioners, NGOs and representatives of local self government besides others are availing this facility of the Centre. Organisation of seminars and workshops on different thrust areas of environmental law all round the year, are a part of the activities of the Centre. The outcomes of the deliberations that are published have richly contributed to the corpus of Environmental Jurisprudence in India. These are being made use of as policy papers and basic reading materials on the subject

Environmental Law Consultancy Services in CEERA is an attempt to meet the longstanding need of different actors involved in environmental management in India. Under this programme, legal advice is being regularly tendered to the governmental agencies involved at different levels of policy making and implementation in environmental law.

1. Asian Development Bank assisted, Development project for 10 Coastal districts of Karnataka: Consultancy service for group of 45 NGOs.

2. Drafting of Bill on constitution of River Bed authority in Karnataka: Consultancy service for Ministry of Major Irrigation Government of Karnataka.

Projects

The Centre has undertaken an "Environment Management Capacity Building Project (Law Component)" on behalf of the Ministry of Environment and Forests, Government of India. Spread over a period of five years and assisted by the World Bank, the project is expected to produce competent leaders to manage the destiny of India's environment. It has also completed short assignment for Indira Gandhi.

Working in close co-operation with UNEP, UNITAR, IUCN and APCEL, the Centre, with its rich resource base and documentation, is poised to blossom into an Environmental Law Academy for the entire SAARC Region, in the years to come.

Case studies: CEERA has constituted number of case studies based on Doctrinal Legal Research, based on empirical data. The main objective of the case studies is to systematically analyze and understand the Environmental problems in various regions of the country and to find adequate legal solutions. The case studies will add legal value and help in the creation of new knowledge, while dealing with hotspot problem solving. The case studies constituted are on the following areas.

1. Deforestation in the Western Ghats
2. Underground Water table depletion in Mysore and Mandya
3. Lake degradation in Bangalore
4. Documentation of Self Imposed Rules in Uttraranchal
5. River Pollution in Tunga and Bhadra
6. Eco Tourism and development

7. Urbanisation, Industrialisation and Globalisation
8. Salt Water Intrusion in coastal Karnataka.

A Report on the Activities of CEERA (May- July)
Workshop on "Peoples' Participation in Environmental Management, Exploring the Legal Spaces", 15th and 16th May 1999, NLSIU, Bangalore

The Workshop mainly discussed the scope available for public participation in the existing legal order, the legal hurdles to facilitate popular involvement in environmental management, the manner in which the tools and techniques are to be evolved for ensuring democratisation of decision - making processes, participatory monitoring of violations and responsible resource management and the manner in which voluntary organisations and social movements could hasten the process of democratic decentralisation of environmental administration. In order to discuss the above mentioned issues, four broad themes were identified, *viz,* 1) bio-diversity related laws, 2) pollution - control laws, 3) land related laws and 4) laws governing the local self government institutions. The Workshop brought together a cross section of people, predominantly from Bangalore, experts in their own fields committed to the idea of ensuring popular participation at all levels of the decision-making process. The deliberations were fruitful and it was agreed that future meetings to evolve strategies for effective people's participation need to be convened.

Workshop for Industrial Managers on "Compliance with Environmental Law", 29th and 30th May 1999, NLSIU

The objective of the workshop was two fold: to discuss the needs of industrial managers for capacity building and to discuss some of the procedural aspects of environmental law implementation. The Workshop also aimed to provide an opportunity to Industrial Managers to know the law better and the enforcement authorities to be sensitised to the problems faced by the industries. The methods of industrial setting, industrial safety, industry and infrastructure, cleaner production and the updating of the legal capacity of the Industrial Managers were also discussed in the process.

ASC Programme:

Under the World Bank Project on Environmental Law Capacity building in India, CEERA, NLSIU is organising a 21 days ASC Programme in Environmental Law in Bangalore. The programme is essentially aimed at young law teachers at the undergraduate and/or postgraduate level in law teaching institutions. The programme would equip the teachers in teaching environmental law. Some selected teachers will then be given advanced training in Environmental Law both in India and abroad. Application and details of the same are available at ASC Inquiry, CEERA, National Law School of India University, P.B. No. 7201, Nagarbhavi, Bangalore 560 072.

Under the World Bank Project on Environmental Law Capacity building in India, CEERA, NLSIU wants to build partnerships with some law institutions all over the world. By this CEERA would not only build the environmental law capacity in these institutions but would also be aided in efficiently executing the project. Letters of Interest are invited from interested universities. Details about the same are available with, The Partner Institutions Inquiry, CEERA, NLSIU, P.B. No. 7201, Nagarbhavi, Bangalore - 560 072.

CHILIKA

Chilika is charged by the renewed protest regarding the rights of traditional fishermen *vis-a-vis* prawn culture of non-traditional fishermen. The result is the killing of four persons including a woman in Surana village in a clash between both the groups on May 29th. The conflict has reached a climax and the traditional fishermen are demanding a total ban on prawn culture in Chilika and removal of prawn gheries from the lagoons. Chilika provided livelihood to about one and half lakh people (both fishermen and non-fishermen living in and around Chilika in about 132 villages. The 1991 policy of the State Government conferring powers on the District Collector to lease out culture source of fishery to the non fishermen is the major bone of contention between the fishermen community and others. The aforesaid policy is alleged to be the cause of increasing mafia raj in the Chilika Lake area. Prawn culture has mushroomed in these areas owing to the 1991 policy decision. Recently the traditional fishermens community has started demolishing the prawn gheries of the non traditional community as it affects their long term interest. The Matsyajini Mahasangha has asked the State Government to establish a Development Authority for Chilika. The main issues in this recent fight are (a) Does Chilika belong to the inhabitants of Chilika or to the Government? (b) What is the primary concern of the State to save the Chilika ecology by extending protection to the right of traditional fishermen or to protect the non traditional fishermen? This latest round of clashes may well be the beginning of the end of the controversy.

The best possible course of action would be to think of Chilika minus the prawn price tag. The State Government must ensure the compliance of the Supreme Court's decision in S.Jagannath v. Union of India, (1997 2 SCC 87). In that case Court in its order had instructed that no aquaculture activity should be permitted within one kilometer from the Chilika lake.

Induction Training Programme for the Environmental Officers of Karnataka State Pollution Control Board between 14th and 18th June 1999, at NLSIU

Acting upon its mandate under the Capacity Building Project and also upon the request made by the Karnataka State Pollution Control Board, CEERA conducted an induction training programme for the new recruits to the State Pollution Control Board. The main objective of the training programme was to make the officers, (who were mainly from the environmental sciences background), aware of law and legal issues which would help them perform their duties effectively. Topics covered in the training programme included principles of natural justice, the right to information, national environmental policies (including policy on forest and wildlife), relationship between pollution control laws and other related enactments.

Workshop on "Coastal Regulation Zone Notifications and Implementation", 3rd July 1999, S.D.M. Law College, Mangalore

The Workshop was organised to enable Government Officers to familiarize themselves with the CRZ Notification and its implementation and to identify areas of possible co-operation and co-ordination between different departments of the Government. The Workshop was attended by senior dignitaries of the Karnataka Government including Shri S.K. Pattanyak, Secretary, Government of Karnataka and Mr. Shivalingaiah, Chairman, KSPCB. 'Cases and Materials Concerning the Coastal Environment', a publication of CEERA was released at the Workshop. It also strengthened the link with S.D.M. Law College, a potential partner institution.

Because of the rapid growth of Internet resources in all the fields, to scope for legal research has also increased. Large number of legal information available at this web site and the required information can be easily downloaded. This web site is a comprehensive, interactive environmental law internet resource for environmental lawyers, corporate counsel and environmental compliance managers, providing direct access to environmental laws, state, international and tribal, court and environmental agency decisions, documents and databases, and task-specific environmental law libraries. Environmental Law Net also provides valuable environmental law news, environmental law articles, interviews, information, and environmental law research tools for environmental lawyers. (Reference: B.E. Pushpa Kadam Calendar of Events July-September 1999)

ENVIRONMENTAL MANAGEMENT AND POLICY RESEARCH INSTITUTE, BANGALORE EMPRI – News Letter

Environmental Management and policy Research Institute is a Research Institute placed in Bangalore. Its main objectives include, Trainings on Bio-Medical Waste management, Coastal Pollution and its Management, Water and Ground Water Pollution, Natural Resource Exploitation, Land and Sand Pollution, Municipal Solid Waste Management, Pollution Control Laws and Compliance, Bio-Diversity and other environment related issues. It also offers some short term courses on Integrated Environment Management for Government Institutions and Industries, a whole lot of environmental management issues.

- Presently it is conducting few training programmes sponsored by KUIDFC to train local bodies, industries and other stakeholders
- Another training programme on Bio- Medical Waste Management is being conducted in sponsorship with Department of Ecology and Environment, Government of Karnataka to train representatives of Health Care Establishments
- Training on Municipal Solid Waste Management for local bodies
- Rain Water Harvesting
- Bio-Diversity Conservation
- It also organizes Seminars on related issues

EMPRI has completed the work on preparation of Guidelines for environment impact assessment for Sujala

Watershed Project in Karnataka funded by the World Bank. The guidelines developed include the methodology and tools to undertake EIA for watershed activities by the various stakeholders including the communities. EMPRI has also trained Sujala Watershed stakeholders on the use of the guidelines.

The ENVIS node on "Capacity Building for Environment Management" is sponsored by the Ministry Of Environment and Forests, Government of India, under Environment Management Capacity Building Technical Assistance Project (EMCBTA) of the World Bank.

CLIMATE CHANGE CELL AT EMPRI:

Karnataka is one of the rapidly developing states in the country in the areas of industrial and infrastructural development facing environmental stress due to various types of pollution. The state is climatologically very diverse and has the dubious distinction of having the largest area under arid and semi-arid condition. The state has very rich forests with very high biological diversity facing degradation threats due to anthropogenic and other factors.

The state has very large population living below poverty line depending on the natural resources for sustenance and is vulnerable to any climactic change impacts. Recently the state has witnessed series of natural calamities such as drought, floods, depletion of ground water reserve, rising temperature, vegetation wilting, etc. The natural calamities though can be attributed to climatic changes the impacts on the natural resources, health, vegetation, ground water recharge and livelihood systems are quite significant affecting the water resources, crop production, forest resources, bio-diversity, people and related developmental activities.

In this background, it is proposed to initiate some activities to understand the climatic changes impact on the state and to develop some strategic action plan to mitigate the impacts. Some of the activities the climate change cell proposes to address are as follows.

- To act as nodal agency in the state to coordinate the work
- To initiate some studies and survey on the climate change agenda
- To organize workshops and seminars on various themes of climate change to create awareness among the policy makers and other stakeholders
- To create data base on the climate change impacts on various natural resources
- Capacity building
- Monitoring the climate change impacts in the state periodically by establishing base line data
- To develop strategic action plan to mitigate climate change impacts
- To establish networking agencies and individuals working in the field
- To develop projects for GEF and international funding on climate changes
- To provide technical support to the field agencies to prepare projects on carbon sequestration, bio-diversity conservation, GHH gases mitigation, etc.

EMPRI in collaboration with National Institute of Technology, Suratkal & College of Fisheries, Mangalore has organised a national Workshop on "Pollution Impacts on Coastal Ecosystem of Karnataka" during March11-12, 2004 at NITK, Suratkal. The Workshop was inaugurated by Prof. B. Hanumaiah, Vice Chancellor, Mangalore University and attended by researchers from various institutions, officers from various Government Departments; NGOs and others. The Workshop was sponsored by the Department of Forest, Ecology & Environment, Government of Karnataka,

Karnataka State Pollution Control Board & Karnataka Urban Infrastructure Development & Finance Corporation, Government of Karnataka.

KARNATAKA STATE POLLUTION CONTROL BOARD (KSPCB)

KSPCB has organised THUNGABHADRA, An Exhibition on Environment for Industries. The Components of this mobile exhibition are:

- General Features of Karnataka
- Industries and their contribution
- Small-scale industries in Karnataka
- Problems of Small-scale industries
- Resource Depletion and Environmental pollution
- Major pollutants of selected Small-scale industries
- Occupational Health Hazards
- Water Quality Standards
- pH Metre
- Dissolved Oxygen Metre
- Sound Level Metre
- Simple Educational Interactive activities like, district-wise distribution of Small-scale industries in Karnataka (Mar-2001), revolving display board, industrial safety devices, illustrative display of Air, Water, Sound and Solid Waste Pollution.
- Environmental concerns of Sericulture Industry
- Rain Water Harvesting in Industry
- Electroplating-pollution Control Mechanism
- Effluent Treatment Plant
- Boiler-pollution Control Mechanism
- Cupola (Foundry) Pollution Control Mechanism

FOUNDATION FOR NATURAL EXPLORATION AND ENVIRONMENTAL CONSERVATION (NEC)

Objectives: NEC was found in 1992 with a view to;

- Encourage and propagate conservation of environment for sustainable development
- Facilitate and promote environmental information networks
- Promote exploration of nature to enhance nature awareness

Activities:

- Organising seminars, workshops, camps, field-visits, etc. to propagate and stimulate conservation of nature
- Rendering professional services tin organising and conducting Environmental related programmes
- Providing expert assistance to various projects
- Assisting in publication of books and reports
- Organising special programmes for exploring the nature

Current activities

- Environmental education to students – NEC organizes a variety of activities for students; as they are one of the main target groups, with a view to promote non-curriculum environmental education. NEC is the nodal agency for the implementation of 'Kids for Tigers' programme conducted by Sanctuary Asia and Britannia
- Lakes (Wetlands) – NEC has been involved since 1987 with the study and conservation of wet lands. NEC over the years has built data on lakes in and around Bangalore. NEC has also been coordinating activities of the 'Inland Wetlands of India' – a conservation plan for wetland protected areas, under a project implemented by the Salim Ali Centre for Ornithology and Natural History (SACON), Coimbatore

- Nature exploration – Eco adventure
- Research & Information dissemination

SAMAGRA VIKAS

Bangalore December 31: Samagra Vikas, an organisation working in the field of environment and development, has organised a national seminar on "Linking of rivers: Prospects and implications" here on January 4, 2004. Addressing presspersons here on Tuesday, Y.B. Ramakrishna, President, Samagra Vikas, said the seminar, to be held at Kannada Bhavan, would have five sessions. Sri Gangadharendra Saraswathi Mahaswamiji of Swarnavalli Mahasamsthana, Sonda, would inaugurate the seminar which would be attended by 150 people from related fields. P. Majumdar, Associate Professor, Department of Civil Engineering, Indian Institute of Science and a member of the Core Committee of the Task Force on Interlinking of Rivers, would deliver a talk on "Interlinking of rivers: Proposals and realities". Anupam Mishra, Secretary, Gandhi Peace Foundation, New Delhi, would present a paper on "Interlinking of Rivers: A Social perspective", he said. While K.N. Govindacharya, social and political activist, would speak on "Interlinking of rivers: Opportunities and challenges", Keshava Hegde Korse of the Department of Pharmacognacy, S.D.M. College, Ujire, would present a paper on "A case study of linking of Bedthi and Varda rivers". Mr. Ramakrishna said the seminar would conclude with a panel discussion on "Diversion of west-flowing Netravathi river waters to North and East: Is it viable?" Ananth Hegde Ashisara, environmental activist and convener of the Save the Western Ghats Movement, briefed presspersons about the initiatives being taken by environmental groups to educate people about what he said would be the disastrous effects of linking the Bedthi and the Varda. Mr. Hegde said various organisations from across the State such as the Nagarika Seva Trust, Guruvayanakére; Vrikshalaksha Andolan; the Seva Sagar

Trust, Sagar; Bedthi-Aghinashini Kolla Samrakshana Samithi; Uttara Kannada Zilla Parisara Samrakshana Samithi; and Avinasha, Shimoga; would be participating in the seminar.

Efforts by the Association for Tropical Biology (ATB) and the Ashoka Trust for Research in Ecology and the Environment (ATREE) through ATB and ATREE on research priorities for tropical biology began with a discussion by the ATB Council Meeting led President Bawa in Bloomington, Indiana,

1) An opportunity for self-reflection, both individual and collective;
2) Partnerships with other allied organisations;
3) A stronger ATB profile with decision-makers and funding agencies;
4) A set of priorities with strategies to address these priorities and identification of the resources needed to implement those strategies.

DECCAN DEVELOPMENT SOCIETY (DDS)

DDS started as the commitment of a group of professionals to the people of its present project region (Zaheerabad) to continue a rural development project which was abandoned by an industrial house due to its own politico-economic compulsions. The earliest objectives of DDS were to combine ecological and employment parameters to regenerate the livelihoods of the people in the area. It was also transfer of people-oriented technology. Gradually it has evolved into a programme which has three guiding principles: gender justice, environmental-soundness and people's knowledge.

DDS is a grassroots organisation working with Sanghams (village level groups) of poor women most of who are dalits. The societies have a vision of consolidating these village groups into strong and vibrant organs of primary civil society and federate them into a strong pressure lobby for women, poor and dalits. A host of continuing dialogues, debates, educational and training programmes facilitated by the Society with the people tries to translate this vision into a reality.

Alongside this ideological role the Society is also trying to reverse the historical process of degradation of the environment and people's livelihood system in this region through a string of land-related activities like permaculture, community grain fund, community green fund, community gene fund and collective cultivation through land lease, etc. These activities, along side taking on the role of earth care are also resulting in human care by giving the women a new-found dignity and profile in their village communities.

When DDS was founded in 1983, there were six founder members all of who were professionals in various fields : Development Economy, Social Science research, Management Sciences, Communication Technology, Social Anthropology and Development Management. The vision of the society then was to give a leadership to the community groups from outside and facilitate a humane transfer of technology. As the Society grew more people joined from outside: agriculture engineers, permaculturists, foresters, environment scientists, psychologists and feminists, almost everyone from outside.

Slowly as the fascination and curiosity of the outsiders for rural work waned, one after another they withdrew slowly and remained where they belonged : in urban settings, doing what they would do best: management, consultancies, teaching, networking and such other activities.

The gap left in the internal leadership of the Society is slowly being filled by the real stakeholders of the project: the rural people. A large team of farmers, artisans, barefoot agriculture scientists, foresters, watershed specialists, farm engineers, communicators and such other cadres has emerged in DDS. An overarching leadership of some extremely capable women has slowly taken over the day to day management of various activities. They are also acting as a Think Tank for the core management team of the Society.

This is the leadership which is sustainable and long lasting. More and more they have proved that their capabilities are beyond the ordinary imagination of the so called development experts from urban areas. Today these women can negotiate with anyone on any issue: from food security to video production. They have proved their extraordinary mettle in all these fields.

It is on this leadership that the Society will rely more and more. Bringing more and more outsiders is a harrowing task. A lot of energy and time is invested on them. But the call of the new 'globalisation' in development sector becomes irresistible for these people. The huge salaries, professional fees and profiles are so attractive that before one has finished sculpting them, they are gone. This is most unsustainable. Therefore relying on the real stakeholders in rural areas is not only sustainable but also most satisfying. It also challenges the conventional stereotyped thinking on leadership by facilitating a real rural leadership.

Board

Prof G.S. Aurora (Chairperson) One of the founder members of DDS and a distinguished social scientist. He was formerly professor and dean of Sociology of the most coveted university in the country, the Central University of Hyderabad. Dr (Ms) Rukmini Rao (Director), Active in women's movement, Mr M.V. Sastry (Director), One of the founder members of DDS, Prof (Ms) Shanta Sinha (Director), Professor of Social Science at the Central University of Hyderabad, Ms Jamuna (Director), Very active in women's movement, Mr Raghu Cidambi (Treasurer), One of the founder members of DDS, Mr

Jagannanda Reddy (Director), Development worker, Mr P.V. Satheesh (Secretary), One of the founder members of DDS, Mr K.V. Krishnamachari (Member), A distinguished financial analyst, Prof. B. P. Sanjay (Member), Director in Indian Institute of Mass Communications, New Delhi, Ms Akhileswari (Member), Correspondent, Deccan Herald, Andhra Pradesh, Dr. Mazher Hussain (Member) founder of COVA (Confederation of Voluntery Association). Dr Vinod Pavarala (Member), Reader in Communication in Sarojini Naidu School of Communication and Fine Arts at the Central University of Hyderabad.

Table-No. 60 - Knowledge about the NGOs in the area (Non-governmental organisation)

Sl No	Name of the slum	Yes	Per centage	No	Per centage	Total
1	B. Nagar	8	16	42	84	50
2	R. Nagar	16	32	34	68	50
3	P. Palya	2	4	48	96	50
4	A. Nagar	1	2	49	98	50
5	C. Nagar	16	32	34	68	50
All slums		43	17.2	207	82.8	250

The above table tries to bring out the details of Non-governmental organisations operating in the sample slum areas and the knowledge among the residents about their activities. As per the information collected, though there are few NGOs which are operating in these areas, only a small *per cent* of the sample, i.e., 17.2 per cent of them have reported to be aware of the name and activities being taken up by these organisations. The remaining sample of 82.8 per cent has not come in contact with these NGOs. It can be said that the NGOs need to make themselves popular among the localites and should try to reach maximum number of beneficiaries through some common awareness programmes which could include a large gathering at regular frequencies.

Profile of NGO operating in the selected sample slum:

ASHWA RURAL DEVELOPMENT SOCIETY®

ARDS is a voluntary organisation registered under Societies Registration Act XXI of 1860 in the year 1994 on 18th of November. From past six years, the organisation is engaged in various developmental activities pertaining to Education, Environment, Health, Nutrition, Child Labour Eradiation and Rehabilitation, Natural Resource Management, watershed Development, Enlightenment and Empowerment of Women on welfare activities, legal affairs, dowry harassments and other such atrocities on women, Formation and maintenance of Self-Help Groups, Self employment trainings, etc, focusing on the downtrodden urban poor population in general and slum population in general. They are currently operating in slums present in and around Bangalore city urban and also rural taluks of the district.

The Executive Committee has nine members and all of them are from rural background and belong to weaker sections with a thirst to work for the poor and the downtrodden.

The organisation is actively implementing some Government aided projects in assistance with departments like Women Development Corporation, Women and Child Development Department, Karnataka State Social Welfare Advisory Board, Directorate of Municipal Administration, etc. in many slums of the city and also taluks belonging to Bangalore rural district.

Skill Development Training Programmes are conducted to the poor and unemployed women of slums. The beneficiaries are now enabled to get better job opportunities. For example those who were working as helpers in garments are now been taken as tailors which has helped them to increase their income levels and improve their living conditions.

Blood Donation Camps are being organised in the colleges and university, the blood collected is donated to NIMHANS, Bangalore. This has helped many poor and needy to get required blood for their survival.

Thirteen Self-Help groups are formed and maintained in slum areas belonging to Bapuji Nagar, Kaveri Nagar, Kasturba slum and Avalahalli slum in Bangalore city. In slum areas of Dasarahalli CMC, 42 Self-Help groups are formed and maintained by the organisation. The members have been linked to Banks and other NGOs like Myrada for loans to take up income generation activities which have in turn helped them to improve their living conditions.

Entrepreneurship Development Training Programmes for Women are conducted for a period of two months in Bapuji Nagar, Pantharapalya and Ramanagara of Bangalore Rural District. The beneficiaries are trained in the preparation of items like Phenyl, Plain Shampoo, Herbal Shampoo, Pappad, Nutritious Food, Candle, Soap Powder, Soap Liquid, Sabena, Liquid Blue, Pickle, etc. They are being guided and facilitated to start the production and marketing linkages are also provided for the products.

A non-formal School is run for the benefit of school drop-outs, illiterate youth and adults in the slums. The students are provided with free study material and other accessories.

Many awareness programmes and meetings are held with respect to Reproduction and Child Health, Immunisation, Family Planning methods, Hepatitis, Tuberculosis, HIV/AIDS, Cancer, Health and Hygiene, etc. They are actively participating in the Polio Immunisation Programme every year by motivating the public to bring the children to the booths and get immunised on the scheduled dates.

References

1. *A Report on the Activities of CEERA* (May- July) Workshop on "Peoples'. Participation in Environmental Management, Exploring the Legal Spaces," 15th and 16th May 1999, NLSIU, Bangalore.
2. *A Report on the Activities of Karnataka State Pollution Control Board* (KSPCB).
3. Details of Workshop for Industrial Managers on "Compliance with Environmental Law", 29th and 30th May 1999, NLSIU.
4. Environmental Management and Policy Research Institute, Bangalore EMPRI – News Letter ENVIS, Quarterly, September 2003, Volume 1, No. 2.
5. Details of Environmental Support Group, 1996.

CHAPTER VII

ENVIRONMENTAL LEGISLATIONS- A SOCIOLOGICAL PERSPECTIVE

Although the market system ensures profits to producers, and satisfaction to consumers, there is no internalisation of externality and externalisation is caused by the adverse impact of growth. Correctives such as voluntary bargain, the polluter-pays principle, taxes and subsidies, or even an *ex post* liability approach, have their own limitations in the internalisation of the externalities. Thus, there is a need for state intervention to internalize the externality. Indian courts (the liability system), however, adopted a unique approach of public interest litigation to safeguard public interest against the vested interests.

The law and economic literature has focused on the role of the legal institutions and common law rules in achieving efficiency and distributive goals (Calabresi, 1970; Landes and Posner, 1987; Shavel, 1987) particularly in the area of environmental policy (Polinsky, 1980; Landes and Posner, 1984; Tietenberg, 1989; Kronhauser and Revesz, 1994). This is an *ex post* approach where parties pay damagers after the harm has occurred. Under this approach, courts set the due level of care based on the nature and facts of the case, if harm occurs. On the other hand regulation is an ex *ante* approach, where parties pay a fine after violating regulatory standards, sometimes even before harm has occurred. Standards are defined by the state, which also plays a major role in the enforcement of laws.

There is an overlapping between the liability and regulatory approaches to environmental protection. On the one hand, compliance with regulatory standards does not automatically relieve the party from liability but, on the other hand, non- compliance with regulatory standards does not necessarily make it liable. It may therefore be necessary to use an optimal mix of these two systems, using them as substitutes and complements to correct the externalities.

In the case of joint use of liability and regulation, courts should use a tort liability as a temporary substitute for regulation, when regulation appears to be inefficient. After the correction by regulatory measures, courts should resolve the conflict between *ex ante* and *ex post* approaches. Thus the optimal mix of alternative legal system is one where regulatory authorities set the maximum standards and courts take into consideration these standards and award damage compensation, since the regulatory standards are insufficient to internalize the risk of harm. Similarly the minimum standards of regulation may perhaps reduce the risk of harm in the event that the liability system is unable to do so. Thus, the optimal mix of liability and regulation should provide incentives to the parties to take precautionary measures in order to reduce the risk of harm.

Environmental law

The Indian constitution provides for power sharing between the union and state governments. Parliament has the power to legislate for the whole country, while the state legislatures are empowered to make laws only for their respective territorial jurisdictions. Under Article 246 of the Constitution, the subject areas of legislation are divided between the union and the states into three lists, union, state and concurrent list. Central law prevails over state law in the concurrent list, however state law prevails if it has received presidential assent. The Constitution also provides that the centre may enact laws on the state list, after receiving consent from the respective states.

After the 1972 UN conference on Environment and Human Development at Stockholm, the Indian government incorporated Articles 48A, Article 51A (g), and 253, to the Indian Constitution. On the basis of these articles, parliament enacted the Prevention and Control of Pollution Act, 1981 (Air act), and the Environmental Protection Act of 1986.

Environmental legislation in India:

(1) The water Act of 1974 (Amendment, 1988): This is the first law passed in India whose objective was to ensure that domestic and industrial pollutants are not discharged into rivers and lakes without adequate treatment. The reason is that such a discharge renders the water unsuitable for drinking, irrigation and to support marine life.

In order to achieve its objective, pollution control boards at the central and state levels were created to establish and enforce standards for factories discharging pollutants into bodies of water. The state boards are empowered to issue consent for establishment (CFE) wherever a firm wanted to establish a new factory and also issue consent for operation (CFO) for existing factories. They were also given the authority to close factories or, in the case of disconnecting power and water supply, issue directions to the concerned departments for enforcement of board's standards.

(2) The Air Act of 1981 (Amendment, 1987): The objective of the Air Act of 1981 was to control and reduce air pollution. The working of this act and the enforcement mechanisms are similar to that of the Water Act. What was novel was that the act also called for the abatement of noise pollution.

(3) Environmental Protection Act, 1986 (The EP Act): The objective of the EP Act is to protect and improve the environment in the country. It is an umbrella legislation that consolidated the provisions of the air and water acts. Environmental disasters prodded the Indian government into passing comprehensive legislation, including rules relating to storing, handling and use of hazardous waste.

The EP Act empowered the Indian government to make rules and regulations to fulfill its objectives. Under this Act and its rules the government takes all necessary steps, such as the formulation of national environmental standards, prescribe procedures for managing hazardous substances, regulate industrial locations, establish safeguards for preventing accidents, and collect and disseminate information regarding environmental pollution. It also empowered the government to set up parallel regulatory agency to protect parts of the environment and to delegate its powers to such an agency to protect coastal resources.

The EP Act provided for civil and criminal penalties for the violation of its pollution standards. For example, it imposes a penalty for non-compliance of standards with a fine of up to Rs 1,00,000 or imprisonment up to five years, or both.

(4) The Product Liability Insurance Act, (1991): The focus of this act was to provide for the payment of immediate compensation to the victims of industrial accidents.

Enforcement of Environmental Laws

Environmental laws are enforced not only by pollution control board set up at federal and state levels, but also by the Supreme Court and the High Courts of respective states through a process called public interest litigation (PIL). Before describing the use of PIL, it is instructive to learn about the structure of the Indian judicial system.

Supreme Court: The Supreme Court is the apex court that has both original and appellate jurisdiction. It is under this article that the court initiated the concept PIL which is unique to the Indian court system. Under it, any individual or group of individuals can ask the court for relief against the actions or the lack thereof of the government or its agencies. The court issues a writ of mandamus ordering the government or its agencies to perform its duties that are mandated by the law.

High Courts: The High Court is the apex court of every state of the Indian Union and is constituted under the provisions of the Indian Constitution. It, too, has writ jurisdiction under Article 226 of the Constitution.

PIL and the Indian courts: The Indian liability system adopted PIL to safeguard the public at large by increasing its accessibility. Under the provision of the PIL, a letter to the courts could be treated as a petition. The courts even provide legal aid to argue the case on behalf of the petitioner. The concept of PIL was initially adapted by Krishna Iyer in 1976 (without assigning the terminology) in the Mumbai Kamgar Sabha v/s Abdulbhai. In fact the terminology 'public interest litigation' was used in Fertilizers Corporation Kamgar Union v/s Union of India. However, the concept took roots firmly in the Indian judiciary in S.P.Gupta v/s Union of India.

Courts and environmental PIL: We focus on the use of the court system and the writ jurisdiction of the Supreme Court and High Court to enforce laws to improve environmental quality in the country. We study all cases filed in the Supreme Court and the High Court.

Few examples of the courts decisions have been included in this chapter to illustrate the pivotal role that Public Interest Litigation plays in the field of environmental protection. Discussion in the previous chapter shows clearly that environmental protection has become a social movement. Given the magnitude of environmental changes and the serious health problems that inevitably follow, not to speak of down-to-earth struggle over the resources that people have responded overwhelmingly, environmental protection is therefore a major challenge. The legislation, the bureaucracy and the judiciary and the civil society are involved each in its own way in this gigantic task. The role of State or Government, the Courts and the civil society in terms of environmental movement has been discussed to show the stakes involved and the stakeholders.

We have inherited a system of colonial rule and we have continued the culture. As a result, we do not have a participatory model of standardisation and administration. Naturally, the rule enforcement becomes a top-down model. Though it is easier to build up this capacity in governance, a real capacity is one where people have participation in the rule - making, administration is aware of contemporary needs including the domestic needs and global expectation and the judiciary is competent to respond to system - structure as soon as there is an interest conflict.

All the other stake holders like industries, forest management ecology administration, LSGs, University faculties have to allocate and therefore necessarily have the capacity to allocate human resources to build up capacity for environmental justice. The justice here is not something to be done from the public point of view the apex court but from the point of view of the recipient. A thing which looks exemplary from the top may not see the light of day at the bottom and there lies the test of capacity building. We are now at the juncture from where we have to take off.

References

1. The Water Act of 1974 (Amendment, 1988).
2. The Air Act of 1981 (Amendment, 1987).
3. Environmental Protection Act, 1986.
4. The Product Liability Insurance Act (1991).

CHAPTER VIII

JUDICIAL ACTIVISM AND ENVIRONEMENTAL MANAGEMENT

This chapter studies the use of public interest litigation by the Supreme Court and the Andra Pradesh High Court to improve environmental quality in India. It also provided some case studies (Case study material is reproduced from the Supreme Court judgments). Using a data set of all environmental quality cases filed and disposed in the Supreme Court for the years 1990 to 1999, we find the exercise of writ jurisdiction by these courts helps in improvement of environmental quality. There are however many important qualifiers both in decisions made by these courts and in the implementation of their orders. We find that variables like a visit by the court to the polluted site, time taken to decide the case and implementation of the order play a positive role in explaining the improvement of environmental quality.

Public Interest Litigation (PIL) and Environmental Protection:

Case Studies (Few Samples)

1. Wing Commander Utpal Barbara & Others v/s State of Assam & Others (AIR 1999 Gauhati 78)

This case was filed under Article 226 of the Constitution of India for issuance of an appropriate writ to quash the order of the Additional District Magistrate banning the use of polythene bags throughout the District of Karnrup in

Assam. The petitioners in this case were the proprietors of factories for manufacturing and supply of polythene bags. They alleged that the order of the Additional District Magistrate under section 144 of the Code of Criminal Procedure had curtailed their fundamental right to carry on trade and business. In the petition they also contended that they had obtained licenses/no objection certificates from the Gauhati Municipal Corporation, District Industries and the Central and State Pollution Control Board. The main issue before the court was whether the Additional District Magistrate had exceeded his jurisdiction under section 144, Cr.P.C. in passing the impugned order banning the use of polythene bags. The Gauhati High Court in its order held that unregulated and indiscriminate use of the polythene bag and its impact on environmental degradation could not be a ground for invoking S. 144, Cr.P.C. by imposing total ban on its use. The single judge bench also made it clear that if the district administration or the State Government considered that a total ban of polythene bag use was required, they could impose it by taking resort to appropriate legislations. The court also categorically pointed out that in the above mentioned facts S.144 Cr.P.C. could be used for a short period but not in perpetuity.

2. The Goa Foundation & Another v/s The Conservator of Forest; Forest Department, Panaji, Goa & Others. (AIR 1999 Bombay 177)

A Public Interest Litigation was filed by the Goa Foundation challenging the permission granted by the Conservator of Forests contrary to the Forest (Conservation) Act 1980 for carrying our certain developmental activities in the forest area of village Penha de Frana of Bartez Taluka of Goa. According to the petitioner, the land in question was a forest land and non forest activity therein was not permissible unless prior permission was taken from the Central Government under the Forest Conservation Act 1980. The petitioner alleged that alterations were made in the survey record for facilitating the residential complex work in the area of 11.275 sq metres. The Court looked into the rival contentions made by the Forest Department by scrutinising the past record of the land. It also verified the Forest Department instructions for application of Forest (Conservation) Act 1980 to private forest. Tracing the history of the said land the court observed that the construction activity in these areas was for a non-forest purpose and as no approval had been taken from the Central Government in this regard the developmental activity carried out in the area had to be stopped.

3. Mukul Roy v/s State of Ors (1999(1) CHN 585)

The petitioner, the General Secretary of All India Trinamul Congress filed this writ petition praying for cancellation of the election programme in two districts of Darjeeling or to reschedule the Madhyamik and Higher Secondary Examination (as the same was scheduled at the time of election) and alternatively for making suitable relaxation of the ban on use of loud speakers and microphones during the examination period for facilitating the election campaign. It was argued by the petitioner that as the election process had already commenced there was no scope for deferring the election. The respondents also contended that the examinations could not be rescheduled. So the Court was left with the option of considering the co-existence of both the programmes keeping in mind the impact of sound pollution on the environment. In the light of the above mentioned circumstances the Court ordered a total ban on the use of microphones in any residential or mixed residential area and within half a kilometer of such area where the examination was due. It also made clear that microphones fitted with sound limiters could however be used for the purpose of election propaganda outside such area only from 5 p.m. to 7 p.m but maintaining a sound limit not exceeding 45 dB and not affecting the silence zone.

4. M.C. Mehta v/s Union of India and Others (Interim Order) (Order dated April 16th, 1999, April 29th 99 and order dated May 13th, 99)

Keeping in mind the vehicular pollution in Delhi in the next millennium, a Public Interest Litigation was filed by Mr. M.C. Mehta in the Supreme Court of India seeking various reliefs from the court to curb the vehicular traffic in Delhi. On 7th January 1998 a committee had been constituted under the Chairmanship of Sri Bhure Lal known as "Environment Pollution (Prevention and Control) Authority for the National Capital Region and a direction was issued by the apex court to submit a report about the action taken by the committee for controlling vehicular pollution and matters connected therewith. As per its order, dated April 16th, the Court perused the report submitted by the said committee (of April 1, 1999). According to the report private (non commercial vehicle comprise 90 per cent of the Nitrogen Oxide (NOx) and respirable particulate matter (RSPM) from vehicular exhaust over Delhi is due to diesel emission. It was estimated that chronic exposure to such toxic air contaminant would lead to 300 additional cases of lung cancer per year. The petitioner has prayed before the court to suspend the registration of diesel vehicles in Delhi until further orders are passed by the court as the automobile industries sought time for examining the proposal made by others with regard to Euro norms. When the matter came up for hearing on April 29th considering the suggestions made by Bhure Lal Committee, Amicus Curie and automobile manufacturers the court forced the Indian Automobile Industries to confirm to the Euro II and Euro III norms. The court in its order directed all private (non commercial) vehicles which conforms to Euro II norm to be registered in the NCR without, restriction. All private (non commercial) vehicles shall conform to Euro I norm by 1st June, 1999. The same type of vehicle shall conform to Euro II norms to 1st April 2000. This direction will be applicable to diesel and petrol driven cars (private non commercial vehicle). To facilitate registration the court further observed the registering authority may register the vehicle concerned on a certificate of the manufacture duly authenticated by the authorised officer certifying that the vehicle concerned confirm to Euro I/Euro II norms. In its 13th May order the court clarified that restriction imposed on April 29th order would not apply to registration of vehicles which are fitted with Compressed Natural Gas (CNG) kits and ply on CNG only. It is also clarified in this order that Euro I norm for the purpose has been notified by the Government of India through a Notification dated 28.8.97.

5. Public Health

Public Health law imposes various duties on local authorities. It is essentially local in character and is easily available for use by private citizens, though is hardly ever used. Article 47 of the Constitution of India makes it a paramount principal of governance that steps be taken for the improvement of public health. A citizen can also evoke Article 51 A (g) for the enforce-ment of duties cast on State instrumentalities, agencies, departments, local bodies and statutory authori-ties. It is the duty of the municipality to remove the filth and rubbish from its municipal limits. It is also their duty to keep and maintain public streets, places and sewers clean. For this purpose muni-cipal Acts have been enacted which set out the duties and obligations of the municipality towards the public. Section 133 of the Cr. Pc. enables the magistrate to pass orders against individuals, statutory bodies and others to remove the nuisance from a particular area. Filth and insanitary conditions have been held to constitute a nuisance. The courts have also been hard-hitting towards the lacksadaisical and indifferent approach of the Municipality in maintaining the city clean. Local authorities have moved into action only after cases have been filed against them. In Municipal Council, Ratlam

V/s. Vardhichand and Ors (AIR 1980 S.C. 1622), the Municipality approached the Supreme Court for setting aside the order of the Magistrate passed under section 133 of the Cr. Pc, which directed the Municipality to abate the nuisance by covering the drains and removing the dirt and filth. The Supreme Court, however, strongly reprimanded the Municipality for failing to carry out its statutory duties under the Municipal law. It upheld the Magistrate's order stating that the Municipality can not turn its face from its principal duties of preserving public health on the ground that it did not have sufficient funds. The Municipality is bound to maintain the Municipal area clean. Providing public latrines and workable drainage system to meet the needs of the people is the statutory duty of the Municipality.

In L.K. Koolwal Vs. State of Rajasthan (AIR 1988 Rajasthan 2) it was held by the Jaipur Bench of the Rajasthan High Court that maintenance of health, preservation of sanitation and environment falls within the purview of Article 21 since it adversely affects the life of citizens. In this case the residents of Jaipur moved the High Court in the matter of proper sanitation of Jaipur City. The Court held that it was the primary duty of the Municipality to remove filth, rubbish, night soil or any other noxious or offensive matter irrespective of whether it had the funds or not. Thus, an individual can directly file a writ petition in the High Court under Article 21 for adversely affecting their right to life and under Articles 47 and 51A (g) of the Constitution of India to enforce the municipality and other statutory bodies to carry out its duties.

A civil suit can also be filed against the municipality and other statutory bodies praying for a mandatory order directing the authorities to remove the dirt and filth. A criminal complaint under section 133 Cr. PC can be filed against the authorities directing them to remove the nuisance. The magistrate also has powers to pass injunction orders restraining the parties from continuing the nuisance.

Any violation of the orders of the magistrate can be visited with punishment.

6. M.c. Mehta and Another Petitioners

V/S

Union of India and Others Respondents

AND

Sriram Foods and Fertilizer Industries and Another Petitioners

V/S

Union of India and Others Respondents

(P.N. BHAGWATI, C.J. AND D.P. MADON AND G.L.OZA, JJ)

P.N. BHAGWATI, C.J

1. This Writ Petition, which has been brought by way of public interest litigation raised some seminal questions concerning the true scope and ambit of Articles 21 and 32 of the Constitution, the principles and norms for determining the liability of large enterprises engaged in manufacture and sale of hazardous products, the basis on which damages in case of such liability should be quantified and whether such large enterprises should be allowed to continue to function in thickly populated areas and if they are permitted so to function, what measures must be taken for the purpose of reducing to a minimum the hazard to the workmen and the community living in the neighbourhood. These questions which have been raised by the petitioner are questions of the greatest importance particularly since, following upon the leakage of MIC gas from the Union Carbide Plant in Bhopal, lawyers, judges and jurists are considerably exercised as to what controls, whether by way of relocation or by way of installation of adequate safety devices, need to be imposed on Corporations employing hazardous technology and producing toxic or dangerous substances and if any liquid

or gas escapes which is injurious to the workmen and the people living in the surrounding areas, on account of negligence or otherwise, what is the extent of liability of such Corporations and what remedies can be devised for enforcing such liability with a view to securing payment of damages to the persons affected by such leakage of liquid or gas. These questions arise in the present case since on December 4 and 6, 1985 there was admittedly leakage of oleum gas from one of the units of Shriram Foods and Fertilizer Industries and as a result of such leakage, several persons were affected and according to the petitioner and the Delhi Bar Association, one advocate practicing in the Tis Hazari Courts died. We propose to hear detailed arguments on these questions at a later date. But one pressing issue which has to be decided by us immediately is whether we should allow the caustic chlorine plant of Shriram Foods and Fertilizers Industries to be restarted and that is the question which we are proceeding to decide in this judgment.

2. Delhi Cloth Mills Ltd. is a public limited company having its registered office in Delhi. It runs an enterprises called Shriram Foods and Fertilizers Industries and this enterprise has several units engaged in the manufacture of caustic soda, chlorine, hydrochloric acid, stable bleaching powder, super-phosphate, vanaspati, soap, sulphuric acid, alum-anhydrous sodium sulphate, high test hypochlorite and active earth. These various units are all set up in a single complex, situated, in approximately 76 acres and they are surrounded by thickly populated colonies such as Punjabi Bagh, West Patel Nagar, Karampura, Ashok Vihar, Tri Nagar and Shastri Nagar and within a radius of 3 kilometres from this complex there is population of approximately 2, 00,000. This plant was commissioned in the year 1949 and it has strength of about 263 employees including executives, supervisors, staff and workers. It appears that until the Bhopal tragedy, no one, neither the management of Shriram Foods and Fertilizers Industries

(hereinafter referred to as Shriram) nor the Government seemed to have bothered at all about the hazardous character of caustic chloride plant of Shriram. But, it seems that the Bhopal disaster shook off the lethargy of every one and triggered off a new way of consciousness and every government became alerted to the necessity of examining whether industries employing hazardous technology and producing dangerous commodities were equipped with proper and adequate safety and pollution control devices and whether they posed any danger to the workmen and the community living around them. The Labour Ministry of the Government of India accordingly commissioned 'Technica', a firm of consultants, scientists and engineers of United Kingdom, to visit the caustic chlorine plant of Shriram and make a report in regard to the areas of concern and potential problems relating to that plant. Dr. Slater visited the caustic chlorine plant on behalf of Technica sometime in June-July 1985 and submitted a report to the Government of India summarising the initial impressions formed during his visit and subsequent dialogue with the management and with one Mr. Harries. This report was admittedly not an in depth engineering study but it set out the prelimi-nary conclusions of Dr. Slater in regard to the areas of concern and potential problems. We do not propose to rely very much on this report since it is a preliminary report.

3. It appears that a question was raised in Parliament sometime in March 1985 in regard to the possibility of major leakage liquid chlorine from the caustic chlorine unit of Shriram and of danger to the lives of thousands of workers and others. The Minister of Chemicals and Fertilizers, in answer to this question, stated on the floor of the House that the Government of India was fully conscious of the problem of hazards from dangerous and toxic processes and assured the House that the necessary steps for securing observance of safety standards would be taken early In the interest of the workers and the general public. Pursuant

to this assurance, the Delhi Administration constituted an Expert Committee consisting of Shri Manmohan Singh, Chief Manager, IPCL, Baroda, as Chairman and 3 other persons as members to go into the existence of safety and pollution control measures covering all aspects such as storage, manufacture, and handling of chlorine in Shriram and to suggest measures necessary for strengthening safety and pollution control arrangements with a view to eliminating community risk. The Manmohan Singh Committee visited the caustic chlorine plant and inspected various operations Including storage tanks, cylinders and tonners and obtained detailed information from the management and after a thorough and exhaustive inquiry, submitted its report to the government. This report is a detailed report dealing exclusively with the caustic chlorine plant and considerable reliance must, therefore, be placed upon it. The Manmohan Singh Committee made various recommendations in this report in regard to safety and pollution control measures with a view to minimising hazard to the work-men and the public and obviously the caustic chlorine plant cannot be allowed to be restarted unless these recommendations are strictly complied with by the management of Shriram.

4. Now, on December 4, 1985 a major leakage of oleum gas took place from one of the units of Shriram and this leakage affected a large number of persons, both amongst the workmen and the public, and, according to the petitioner, an advocate practicing in the Tis Hazari Courts died on account of inhalation of oleum gas. The leakage resulted from the bursting of the tank containing oleum gas as a result of the collapse of the structure on which it was mounted and it created a scare amongst the people residing in that area. Hardly had the people got out of the shock of this disaster when, within two days, another leakage, though this time a minor one, took place as a result of escape of oleum gas from the joints of a pipe. The immediate response of the Delhi Administration to these

two leakages was the making of an order dated December 6, 1985 by the District Magistrate, Delhi under sub-section (J) of Section 133 of the Code of Criminal Procedure, directing and requiring Shriram within two days from the date of issue of the order to cease carrying on the occupation of manufacturing and processing hazardous and lethal chemicals and gases including chlorine, oleum, super-chlorine, phosphate, etc. at their establishment in Delhi and within, seven days to remove such chemicals and gases from the said place and not again to keep or store them at the same place or to appear on December 17, 1985 in the court of the District Magistrate, Delhi to show cause why the order should not be enforced. When we took up the writ petitions for hearing on December 7, 1985, our attention was drawn to this order made by the District Magistrate, Delhi on December 6, 1985 and on perusing the order we pointed out the inadequacies in it which had the effect of virtually defeating the urgency of the action to be taken. We had earlier appointed a team of experts to visit the caustic chlorine plant of Shriram and to report whether the recommendations of the Manmohan Singh Committee had been carried out by the management and this team of experts orally reported to us at the hearing on December 7, 1985 that they had been able to inspect the plant for only a couple of hours and that cursory inspection showed that many of the recommendations of the Manmohan Singh Committee appeared to have been complied with and that too two one hundred MT tanks for storage of chlorine which constituted a major element of hazard or risk had been emptied. Since this inspection made by the team of experts had necessarily to be very hurried. and superficial on account of want of sufficient time, we adjourned the writ petition on December 13, 1985, with a direction that the petitioner would be entitled to appoint his own team of experts who would 'be allowed access to the caustic chlorine plant for the purpose of ascertaining whether the various recommendations of the Manmohan

Singh Committee had been carried out or not and whether there were any other drawbacks or deficiencies likely to endanger the lives of workmen and the public. We also, with a view to expediting adjudication of claims for compen-sation on behalf of the victims of oleum gas, leakage, appointed the Chief Metropolitan Magistrate as the officer before whom claims for compensation may be filed by persons affected by leakage of oleum gas in the course of the two incidents referred to above and we fixed time of four weeks within which such claim of compensation may be filed before the Chief Metropolitan Magistrate, Delhi. We may point out that subsequently by an order dated January 16, 1986 we extended the time for filing of compensation claims up to January 31, 1986. We also by our orders dated January 10, 1986 and January 21, 1986 gave a further direction that those who file compensation claims before the Chief Metropolitan Magistrate, Delhi should be got examined by a team of Medical Experts and this task was entrusted to the Secretary of the Delhi State Legal Aid and Advice Board. This direction was given by us with a view to ensuring that contemporaneous medical evidence of the Injuries suffered by the claimants and of the cause of such injury should be avallable In support of the claims for compensation lodged by the victims of oleum gas leakage.

5. Pursuant to the liberty given by us, the petitioner appointed an Expert Committee consisting of Dr. G.D. Agarwal, Professor T. Shivaji Rao and Shri Purkayastha. This committee, which we shall hereafter refer to as the 'Agarwal Committee', visited the caustic chlorine plant and submitted a report to this Court in which it pointed out various inadequacies in the plant and expressed the opinion that it was not possible to eliminate hazard to the public so long as the plant remained at the present location.

6. Since there were conflicting opinions put forward before us in regard to the question whether the caustic chlorine plant should be allowed to be restarted without any real

hazard or risk to the workmen and the public at large, we thought it desirable to appoint an independent team of experts to assist us in this task. We accordingly by an order dated December 18, 1985 constituted a Committee of Experts consisting of Dr. Nilay Choudhary as Chairman and Dr. Aghoramurty and Mr. R.K. Garg as members to inspect the caustic chlorine plant and submit a report to the court on the following three points:

1. Whether the plant can be allowed to recommence the operations in its present state and condition?
2. If not, what are the measures required to be adopted against the hazard or possibility of leaks, explosion, pollution of air and water, etc. for this purpose?
3. How many, of the safety devices against the above hazards and possibility exist in the plant at present and which of them, though necessary, are not instal1ed in the plant?

7. This Committee of Experts to which we shall hereafter, for the sake of convenience, refer to as 'Nilay Choudhary Committee', visited the caustic, chlorine plant on December 28, 1985 and after considering the reports of Dr. Slater, Manmohan Singh Committee and Agarwal Committee and hearing the parties made a report to the court setting out 14 recommendations which in its opinion were required to be complied with by the management in order to minimize the hazards due to possible chlorine leak. Nilay Choudhary CommJttee pointed out that it was in agreement with the recommendations made in the report of the Manmohan Singh Committee which were exhaustive in nature and obviously the recommendations made by it in its report were supplementary recommendations in addition to those contained in Manmohan Singh Committee's report.

8. We have thus two major reports, one of Manmohan Singh Committee and the other of Nilay Choudhary Committee, setting out the recommendations which must be complied with by the management of Shriram in order

to minimize the hazard or risk which the caustic chlorine plant poses to the workmen and the public. The question is whether these recommendations have been complied with by the manage-ment of Shriram, for it is only if these recommendations have been carried out that we can possibly consider whether the caustic chlorine plant should be allowed to be restarted.

9. Since the leakage of oleum gas caused serious public concern, the Lt. Governor of Delhi constitu-ted an Expert Committee consisting of Shri N.K. Seturaman as Chairman and four other experts as members to go into the cause of spillage of oleum and its after-effects, to examine if inspection and safety procedures prescribed under the existing laws and rules were followed by Shriram, to fix responsibility for the leakage of oleum gas, to review the emergency plans and measures for containment of risk in the event of occurrence of such situations and for elimination of pollution, to examine any other aspects that may have a bearing on safety, pollution control and hazard to the public from the factory of Shriram, to make specific recommendations with a view to achieving effective pollution control and safety measures in the factory and to advise whether the factory should be shifted away from its present location in densely populated area. This Committee to which we shall hereafter refer to as the 'Seturaman Committee' made an on the spot inspection of the site of the factory and after obtaining the required information about the plant submitted a report on January 3, 1986. This report must be conceded, deals primarily with the safety procedures in the sulphuric acid plant from which there was oleum gas leakage and is not based on any in depth review and study of safety and pollution control measures in the caustic chlorine plant. But even so it does contain some observations which have relevance to the question whether the caustic chlorine plant poses any hazard to the community and what steps to minimize the risk to the people living in the vicinity.

10. Whilst these proceedings were going on before the Court, order dated December 7, 1985 was issued by the Inspector of Factories, Delhi in exercise of the power conferred under Section 40 sub-section (2) of the Factories Act 1948. the order commenced with the following recital, *viz.*, whereas it has appeared to me that caustic chlorine plant and sulphuric acid plant are running without adequate safety measures being adopted by your management, thereby endangering the human life and safety of the workers and the public at large. Earlier notices of the Labour Department asking your management to ensure safety measures has not been complied with fully; and whereas, in spite of your management's assurance vode letter dated October 14, 1985, on December 4, 1985, non-adoption of the adequate safety measures have resulted in the co11apse of the structure on which oleum tank was mounted resulting in the massive leakage of oleum causing fumes in the environment affecting the health and safety of a large number of residents of the Union Territory of Delhi; and whereas the factory is not still having adequate safety measures required for such plants and prohibited Shriram from using the caustic chlorine and sulphuric acid plants till adequate safety measures are adopted and imminent danger to human life is eliminated. Soon thereafter, on December 13, 1985, a show-cause notice was issued by the Assistant Commissioner (Factories) of the Municipal Corporation of Delhi calling upon Shriram to show as to why action for revocation of its license should not be taken under Section 430 sub-section 3 of the Municipal Corporation Act 1957 for violation of the terms and conditions of the license. Shriram by its letter dated December 23, 1985 showed cause against the proposed cancellation of its license but by an order dated December 24, 1985, the Assistant Commissioner (Factories) directed Shriram to stop Industrial use of the premises at which the chlorine caustic plant is located. The result is that unless these two orders. One dated December 7, 1985 and other

dated December 24, 1985 are vacated or suspended, Shriram cannot be allowed to restart the caustic chlorine plant.

A Review of the sample of Judgments delivered by the highest court of the land under the Public Interest Litigation system shows that environmental protection in a multi-dimensional phenomena and that Supreme Court in particular and High Courts in general have played a vital role in this regard. Indian constitution, the most progressive written document in the world, both in its basic structure and the underlying spirit give utmost significance and concern on issues and problems which impinge upon the public interests and the interests of the common man. Environment issues are inextricably intertwined with social caste and class interests. Conflicts over control, use and own of environmental resources inevitably involves conflicts of interests across a wide-array of castes and classes in India. What is, however, of social concern is the delay and plausible sabotage associated with the process of implementation and monitoring of court decisions. Given the strong environmental movement and a large number of environmental activist groups which we discussed in the previous chapter we are yet to go a long way in breaking the control of vested –interests who are often found hand in glove with the political elites.

Environmental protection continues to remain a formidable challenge of the contemporary society. What is, however, most heartening is the positive response with which civil society has almost always responded to challenges posed by environmental degradation.

The cases have been reproduced almost verbatim from the the judgments given by the courts on PIL (Public Interest Litigation). The author profusely acknowledges the fact that environmental protection is a serious and multidimensional challenge. Wide range of players is involved in this task. All said and done the interventions by the courts has led more often than not in being the veted interests to book. Judiciary has involved itself actively in this task.

References

1. Prasad, P.M., January 17, 2004: (Much of the material has been drawn from) article published in special article, Environmental Protection: The role of Liability System in India, By, Economic and Political Weekly, PP. 257-259.
2. Tripathy, Bibhu Prasad., 2004: 'Public litigation' Environment support Group CEERA (ESG website).
3. The case studies have been drawn from the judgments given by the courts on PIL (Public Interest Litigation).

CHAPTER IX

STATE OF ENVIRONMENT IN FUTURE

Given the serious concern with which environment is looked upon, the present study naturally acquires a phenomenal significance and importance. Slums have come to pose many serious problems in urban communities. Social problems of industrial cities have received the maximum and serious attention of sociologists and social anthropologists. Slums and the environmental degradation is one such serious problem which has so far received hardly any serious attention of sociologists. With a view to examining environmental degradation due to increase in slum population one needs to look at a whole gamut of socio-economic and bio-physical parameters like growth of population, poverty, depletion of the sources, contamination of water, decline in the food security to mention a few examples. At the same time, one needs to examine the dialectical relationship between social life and environment in a holistic perspective.

A) Given lot of myths surrounding our conception of health, different people tend to look at health in different ways. Illness has been defined almost exclusively in terms of the physical manifestations and symptoms if any take a fairly long time before they show up and that health specialists could differ from one another in reading and interpreting the exact meaning of the symptoms. The extent to which symptoms show up depends upon such factors as the type of ailment, age, sex, family background of the patient and a host of environmental factors. Alternately and increasingly in terms of Behavioural sciences, health is defined, "as a person's capacity to carry out one's day-to-day activities with a certain amount of confidence, efficiency and competency". Ideally, health refers to social, psychological, physical, cultural and economic well-being of a person. During the last two decades or so, there has been a growing interest in the preventive possibilities of relationship between peoples' health and features of social and economic environment in which people live. Slum as a social disorganisation, social relations have been the casualties. It has been widely believed that the slum populations are increasingly vulnerable to and might actually carry within themselves a wide-variety of diseases including sexually transmitted diseases. It has been found that permissive nature of family life is slums in the single most important factor responsible for the spread of HIV- positive and lack of personal hygiene and community hygiene seem to be causing a number of communicable diseases spread of malaria in the out-skirts of Bangalore city particularly during rainy season.

B) As seen in the chapters, environment refers to all sorts of surroundings which include material, social and spiritual conditions of living beings. When we consider it at a physical entity, environmental problems are consequences of indiscriminate human interventions. The human causation of environmental problems may be clarified by the difference between natural and environmental catastrophes. Former being a dramatic change of the environment caused by natural process without human interventions and the latter changes that are caused at least partly by human interventions. The three broad categories of environmental problems have been noticed. 1) Exhaustion in the form of the depletion of both renewable and non-renewable resources. 2) Pollution which can be defined as the release of harmful substances into the atmosphere resulting in deterioration in the quality of Oxygen, Water and Soil. 3) Disturbance in the biotic and abiotic aspects of environment due to disruption of symbiotic relationship of man, nature and animal.

C) Slums, Urban environment and Health risks: The most pressing environmental health problems today, in terms of disease, illness, disabilities and even death are associated with poor households and communities in the developing world. In rural areas and in the peri-urban slums of the developing world, inadequate shelter, overcrowding, lack of adequate safe drinking water and sanitation, contaminated food, and indoor pollution are by far the greatest environmental threats to human health. These conditions are further compounded by poor nutrition and lack of education, which make people more vulnerable to, and less able to cope with, environmental threats. The low quality of life has deteriorated which is reflected in unhygienic living conditions and inadequate economic resources. Squalor accompanied by outbreak of diseases, high mortality and morbidity makes slum dwellers not only less productive and become drain on main society. Urbanisation has been extensively researched phenomena. The spatial context of Urbanisation should be considered with reference to the process of formation of metropolitan regions and urbanised areas. The conditions – social, economic, technological, demographic, required for generating and consolidating forces of Urbanisation and modernisation would depend not only on the population size of the urban Centre, but also on the functional character, and growth and history of the urban community. Unplanned growth of cities would, overtime, become centres of squalor, squatter settlements, and slum, irregular and haphazard human settlements. The cumulative effect is urban environmental degradation and destruction of the life on earth. The correlation between industrialisation and Urbanisation has been extensively investigated. Studies have shown that there could be Urbanisation without industrialisation. Urbanisation when happens, the social character of Urbanisation has hardly changed. So much so, that, Indian cities have been dubbed as 'urban villages'. From the point of view of environment namely that rapid growth of population resulted in almost inevitably of course in environmental degradation which in turn accentuated poverty. Poverty has innumerable forms and the form in which it has manifested most is maldistribution of environmental resources, increasing level of malnutrition, inadequate nutrition and the increasing vulnerability of vast mass of population to disease, disability and even starvation and death.

This chapter explores the social background of the sample population with reference to the variables included in the study. Each of these variables and the manner in which they interact with one another has been examined across all the five sample slums. This would help to gain certain insights into the actual behaviour of slum people which would impinge on the environment and consequently certain environmental changes occur. Most changes have been negative. Slum people have been known for engaging themselves almost out of necessity in certain economic activities which are predominantly menial, manual, unskilled, and semi-skilled. Majority of the sample in all the five slums is engaged in manual work and occupation, while far less proportion of the sample reported to have engaged in service occupations like teaching, sales, working at home and government employment to mention a few.

It is widely believed that slum people are illiterates, uneducated and show less inclination towards opportunities to get education. This picture has prevailed, no doubt, for a very long time. It is indeed surprising to note that educational level of lower class and lower caste people has been gradually rising.

Household Income is another variable considered to describe social background. In case of unorganised sector, assessing income is one of the difficult and ticklish issues. It is because not only people in the unorganised sector will have no regular income, but also they have no way of keeping track of their income. Yet this variable cannot be ignored. Income gives us some idea regarding economic status of population. The income has bee grouped into least being less than Rs. 1000 and the maximum being Rs. 10, 000.

In the changed scenario from joint to nuclear families today, we can see maximum *per cent* assuming the role of Head of the family in the age group of 21 to 40. It is also evident from the table that the number of women per 1000 men is 932.32 which very much nearer / equal to the state average as per Census 2001: Average family size is around four (4) members in general. Caste composition is another important and interesting aspect of the sample population. Theoretically and empirically institution of caste has been the most extensively researched aspect of the Indian society. For purpose of analysis various castes in the sample have been divided into Upper castes, Upper middle castes, Middle castes, Lower middle castes and Low caste. One thing that strikes immediately is that almost all castes which are found in wider and main stream society have been reflected obviously though in different *percent*age across the five slums. Yet it could be noted that Brahmins are found in the least number. Religious composition of population has among other things serious implications for social harmony in areas where different proportions of different religious groups are present. Out of the total size of the slum population, expectedly 236 Households belongs to Hindus, 9 Households are of Muslims and 5 Household are of Christians. Except in Rajiv Gandhi Nagar slum, in other slums all the religious groups are represented though in each slum Hindus are preponderant.

Though the slums are very much nearer to the main roads, very few house-holds are near the main roads. No government office is situated near the slums. Often it is said that the slums originate either by the side of a big drainage or in the open space available around the drainage but, very few houses are located near the drainage. There is lack of public toilet facilities in the slums. In general, the houses are constructed of poor quality material, with practically little/no space in between. Living space is one thing that definitely reflects the quality life. Given the cramped extremely congested living space, personal hygiene and genital hygiene are the casualties that render the family members highly vulnerable to sexually related diseases. Inadequate housing stock and poor housing conditions create lot of environmental hazards. Poor families often lack the resources that they are unable to avoid situations which might be degrading of their environment. Poor people in crowded squatter settlements frequently endure inadequate access to safe drinking water. Lack of potable safe drinking water forces them to depend upon and overdraw by over-pumping and depletion of ground water. Personal hygiene, cooking energy sources, waste disposal, garbage disposal, hygiene (personal hygiene), latrine (toilet) facilities, drinking water availability, water source, sanitary facilities, self perception of motive regarding marital relation, inter course, attitude towards sex, contraction of diseases, treatment seeking behaviour, disease burden in slums, etc. have been discussed in detail with backdrop of their responses to specific questions in the interview schedule. In the past two decades the World's urban population has increased by about a billion from 1.35 to 2.28 billion. The bulk of this increase has been (about 60 per cent) in Asia and most of it in the South Asian countries. As per the estimates, urban population is close to 400 million in South Asia. This will increase to 800 million in 20 years. In most South Asian cities, urban infrastructure built slowly over several decades, is already under severe strain with continuous migration from rural areas.

The growing demand for food will place enormous pressure on land and resources. Farmers with small plots will be forced to 'mine' their land by cutting the remaining trees of young age in ecologically destructive practices of crop intensification on marginal land. The increased demand for fuel wood which is the major source of household fuel among the low-income groups of the population has led to further deforestation. This would naturally be accompanied by the associated problem of widespread soil erosion, watershed damage and flooding. Urban areas are particularly prone to this problem, but rural areas are not entirely free from it either. The resultant health hazards include water-borne diseases, respiratory diseases, asthma (especially among the young and the aged) and an increased risk of cancer.

South Asian countries are likely to face many problems of food scarcity in this century. The production will fall short of requirements. According to estimates, India would need 400-500 million tones of food grains by 2050, and the other countries of the region would need about 200 million tones. By 2050 South Asia will need to produce around 650 million tones of food grains.

An Urban Agglomeration is a continuous urban spread constituting a city or town and its adjoining urban outgrowth (OG) or two or more physically contiguous cities/towns together with continuous well recognised urban outgrowths, if any, of such cities/ towns. The phenomenon of rapid Urbanisation in conjunction with industrialisation has resulted in the growth of slums. The sprouting of slums occurs due to many factors, such as, the shortage of developed land for housing, the high prices of land beyond the reach of urban poor, a large influx of rural migrants to the cities in search of jobs, etc. In spite of some efforts by the State Governments/UTs to contain the number of slum dwellers, the growth of slums has been increasing rapidly putting tremendous pressure on the existing urban basic services and infrastructure.

The basic characteristics of the slums essentially remain the same i.e. dilapidated and infirm housing structures, poor ventilation, acute over-crowding, and faulty alignment of streets, inadequate lighting, and paucity of safe g water, water-logging during rains, absence of toilet facilities and non-availability of basic physical and social services. The living conditions in slums are usually unhygienic and contrary to all norms of planned urban growth and are an important factor in accelerating transmission of various air and water home diseases.

The chapter highlights the trends in Urbanisation in India with special reference to Bangalore City. Causes and consequences being origin and growth of slums increase in population and environmental degradation.

The Bangalore City Corporation which has 100 wards within its municipal jurisdiction has a population of 4,292,223 accounting for 75.48 per cent of the total population of Bangalore Urban Agglomeration of which 2,240,956 are males and 2,051,267 are females.

There is also information collected from 2001 Census on urban agglomeration/cities having population of more than one million in India 2001, rural-urban distribution of population-India and States/Union territories 2001, urban agglomerations/towns by class/category: census of India 2001: trends in Urbanisation in India, 1901-1991, identified/estimated slum population of million-plus cities, 1991 & 2001(in million), Urbanisation in Karnataka, Growth of Bangalore City during the last 130 years (1871-2001), ward wise population of the Bangalore city corporation, 2001, slums in Karnataka, 2001,Slum

Population totals in Karnataka, 2001 (Provisional Number of Slums in Cities/towns in Karnataka, 2001, Number of towns by civic Status in Karnataka, 2001, Statement showing the Bangalore City Slums details, Statement showing the Bangalore City Declared Slums detail along with brief notes with a view to facilitate better understanding of the concepts discussed both in the preceding as well as forth coming chapters.

Given the backdrop on Urbanisation and its impact on environment, Pollution, Sources of Urban Air Pollution in India, Vehicular Emissions, Vehicular Growth leading to increase in Pollution, Power Plant and Industrial Emissions, Emissions from other Industries, epidemiology and evaluation of health risks from exposure to particulate matter Health and Socioeconomic Status, In-door Air Pollution, Out-door Air Pollution, Unsafe Drinking Water and Poor Sanitation, Health Effects of Air Pollution, etc. are discussed with reference to studies undertaken in this field as examples.

In recent decades, urban-centres in less-industrialised countries in general and India in particular have experienced unprecedented growth, and mega cities with populations of 10 million or more people have emerged in many countries. In India alone there are four such cities, with three others expected to join the ranks in the next 20 years. Globally, many rapidly growing cities are being overwhelmed by environmental problems, particularly air pollution Mega cities of India are no exception to the global pattern of deteriorating urban air quality. Indian cities are among the most polluted in the world, with concentrations of a number of air pollutants being well above level as recommended by the World Health Organisation. The dearth of data exists across the entire causal chain of risk assessment, from sources of pollution to atmospheric concentrations to human exposures and their health effects. Hardly anything is known about unknown sources that contribute to air pollution. The main categories of urban air pollution sources in India are vehicular emissions, industrial emissions, and fuel use for domestic purposes such as cooking, and a potentially large miscellaneous category, which includes burning of household wastes, emissions from small businesses and cremation grounds. Rapid Urbanisation in India has led to an increase in transportation demand that public transport systems have been unable to meet adequately. Consequently, the use of personal vehicles has increased dramatically. Another key issue in the derivation of emission factors is the quality of fuel used. In the Indian context, the quality of fuel, especially adulteration of gasoline by kerosene, is particularly important, if understudied issue. This problem is almost universal among motorised three-wheeled vehicles (auto-rickshaws), which for the most part are not owned by their operators. Along with a brief note about the state of environment in Banglore city, air Pollution at Trinity circle, K.R. Circle, Anand Rao circle, K.R. Market, Jaya Nagar circle, V.V. Puram Circle, and the Noise pollution caused due to traffic noise which adds to stress levels, which is detrimental to everyone's health has been pointed out. Mention is also made of other elements like the pulveriser which makes too loud a racket for the customers, adding to the decibel level are the loudspeakers, either advertising products or haranguing the public, etc.

After gaining independence in 1947, India embarked on a path of rapid industrialisation in all the major manufacturing sectors—iron and steel, heavy manufacturing, industrial and petrochemicals, and agricultural and paper products. Today, despite its label as a "less-industrialised country," India is heavily industrialised, with a thriving manufacturing sector that until recently was largely indigenous. Mumbai and Delhi are both major industrial Centres with many large and small-scale industries. In addition to being India's financial and commercial capital, Mumbai is also India's most industrialised city.

A number of diseases have been associated with inhalation exposure to airborne PM: respiratory disorders whose effects range from minor symptoms such as coughs and dyspnea to severe ones such as acute respiratory infections (ARI), asthma, and pneumonia, chronic obstructive lung diseases such as bronchitis, cardiovascular disease, tuberculosis, lung cancer, and blindness. In addition, perinatal effects such as stillbirths and low birth weights are also associated with air pollution. However, the health end point that is most clearly defined is death, and many epidemiological studies in developed countries focus on obtaining relationships between mortality rates and ambient levels of pollution. A number of authors, however, argue that exposure to PM is an important determinant of mortality, even when socioeconomic status is taken into account. Half of the world's households use biomass fuels, including wood, animal dung, or crop residues, that produce wide-array toxic particles, carbon monoxide, and other indoor pollutants. Exposure to indoor pollutants can cause or aggravate ARIs, including upper respiratory infections such as colds and sore throats, and lower respiratory infections such as pneumonia. Water Pollution through contaminated water and inadequate sanitation cause a range of diseases, many of which are life-threatening. Despite significant investments in improving water supplies and sanitation over the last 20 years, about 18 *per cent* of the World's population still lacks access to safe drinking water, and nearly 40 *per cent* have no access to sanitation. Loss of water tanks in and around Bangalore city, Spatial Analyses in Bangalore City, Regional-wise Spatial and Temporal Analyses, Water Quality in the tanks of Bannerghatta, Sankey, Madivala, Hebbal, Ulsoor, Yediur, and Kamakshipalya, Waste Management, Bio-Medical Waste, Lethal wastes, E-waste, PC waste, etc. which are the root causes for health hazard leaving toxic taste into the lives of human beings has been dealt with.

The factors helping for maintenance and improvement of environment such as Greenery which improves air quality, protects water quality, provides water availability, stabilizes climate, helps preserving biodiversity, prohibits noise and vibration has been stressed upon so as to bring awareness about the importance and need of the hour to address these aspects much seriously.

Perception, attitude and values among other things, together determine human personality. An analysis of these aspects of the sample of slum population becomes absolutely essential for assessing the role of human Behaviours in the field of environmental protection and environmental management. They need to be educated, motivated, mobilised and organised if necessary trained for a planned, consolidated, collective action. Understanding how a community perceives health risks apparently caused by as polluted water, inadequate drainage, or lack of garbage collection is essential to designing effective programmes to address these problems. Discussion of the analysis of empirical data has shown that human behaviour has much to do with environmental changes and the solution to environmental problems has got to be found in the dynamics of behavioural changes. To bring any changes in the existing situation the understanding of the human beings about becomes important and plays a dominant role in deciding the required changes. Similarly, peoples' perception, attitude, knowledge and environmental consciousness (behaviour), self perception regarding marital relation, self-perception regarding inter-course, attitude towards sex, contraction of diseases, treatment seeking behaviour, knowledge regarding sexually transmitted infection/diseases, knowledge of diseases related to sex, awareness on sexually transmitted infections and diseases (STIs/STDs), HIV/ AIDS awareness, awareness about personal hygiene all these play an important role in determining the level of understanding, views on various health and environmental issues, assessing the knowledge of human beings on the same and to react accordingly to bring about the required changes. In spite of poor and limited knowledge about health and diseases on the one hand, it is surprising to note that many of them are very much familiar about HIV / AIDS which reflects the extent of publicity given to the hazards of that disease.

An attempt has been made through the interview schedule to find out whether any of the family members have ever got sexually transmitted infections or diseases (STIs / STDs) and if so, their reaction to it and the changes brought about in their relationships, the social and economic damage caused to the family particularly to the children, impact on neighbours and the society as a whole by the habit of drinking. Sociologists and Social anthropologists define certain patterns of behaviour which influence environment both negatively and positively. Environmental management strategies have got to be design with a view to curbing and discouraging if necessary punishing human behaviour which might be actually harmful to environment.

In order to get the present picture of the surrounding environment, the kind of trees present in the area, advantages from those plants and trees, pet animals if any, etc. have been considered. This information would reveal the importance given to the trees and plants and also animals which are the part and parcel of our lives from time immemorial. The number of persons per household is decreasing in most countries, which also imply a larger number of households. The result is that on average all individuals are occupying more room and less space is available for functions other than dwellings. Firstly the tradition of different generations living together has decreased and secondly of couples living together has decreased. Empirical research on behaviour which is relevant for the environment mostly shows hardly any correlation between concrete types of behaviour. The reason is that there are no social or psychological criteria primarily determining whether or not behaviour is relevant to the environment. The criteria for characterisation of behaviour are of a physical nature, lying beyond social or psychological categories. Because there is no common human origin, behaviour relevant for the environment cannot be described within one dimension. There are no common origins, only common results (environmental damage) and in general these results are only side effects of human behaviour. Data on public perception of the environmental issues are interesting as an indicator of the attention paid to the environment with in society public opinion time series-data show changing attention and concern, cross-sectional research may indicate significant variation between countries are population group.

Widely called 'new social movements', they are so called because they don't subscribe at least explicitly to any class ideologies and that they are committed to holistic approach to development and that local communities must enjoy the fruits of development. Environmental movements have been the most dramatic and visible social movements in the post-World War period. "Earth Day 1970 is often said to represent the debut of the modern environmental movement." Lack of common theoretical thread in sociological studies of environment has been recognised though rather belatedly. The phenomena of environmental issues have a great deal to do with dynamics of human behaviour. The role of social activist groups occupies an important and significant place in the preservation, conservation and protection of environment and environmental management.

Unabated proliferation of voluntary action group over the last two decades has marked the beginning of environmental movements in India resulting in the Chipko movement, the Appiko movement, the Mitti Bachao

Abhiyan, etc. Needless to add most of these groups have been doing excellent work in mobilising and organising people at the local grass root level. They have been getting good co-operation and support from the media both print as well as electronic not speak of strong support ungrudgingly extended by what has come to be known as Judicial activism (see the previous chapter), intellectuals and environmentally sensitive human rights activist groups. For, conflicts over the preservation, use and control of natural resources almost inevitably often boils down to inter-caste and inter-class conflicts. Environmental degradation in India has almost always followed the misuse and abuse of natural resources by vested interest. Environmental degradation in India has almost always followed the misuse and abuse of natural resources by vested interest. The main agenda of the environmental movements, among much else, is basically three folds- 1) to prevent further ecological destruction. 2) Bring about ecological regeneration. 3) To put environment at the service and control of the people, the people usually being defined as the local communities who live within that environment. NGOs have been playing a vital role in effective and positive organisation of environmental movements. Here, an attempt has been made to furnish the details of some NGOs who are exclusively proactive in this direction and have identified themselves with Environmental Activist Groups. A brief description about their activities with respect to environment and natural resource management is mentioned in this section.

Environmental laws and legislations in India have been the most effective instruments of environmental protection, their enforcement, meaning and significance of Public Interest Litigations (PIL) and its role in environmental protection, to improve environmental quality in India through few case studies (samples) wherein the Petitioners have succeeded in preventing further damage or successfully avoided the damage being caused to the

Environment and otherwise have posed a great threat to the health of the public living within the vicinity of such activities. Yet problems arise basically at the level of implementation and enforcement of environmental laws. For, enforcement of laws directly brings the enforcement agencies in direct confrontation with a wide- array of vested interests which includes very often political elites. Lack of environmental consciousness further makes enforcement of environmental legislation a frustrating experience in the recent past Supreme Court in particular and other Court in general have come to play a very important and vital role in regulating human behaviour in the area of environmental protection. Case studies discussed in the chapter mostly drawn from the Supreme Court judgment has served to establish the fact that Judiciary in India has shown an exemplary courage in breaking the control of vested interest and in ensuring environmental justice. Not only the interests of the common man are protected but even the interests of the future generation are protected.

BIBLIOGRAPHY

Agarwal, S.P. 1993: *Impacts of dust pollution*. Indian Journal, Environmental Protection.

Aggarwal, A.L., Raiyani C.V., Patel PD, Shah, P.G., Chatterjee, S.K. 1982: Assessment of exposure to benzo (*a*) pyrene in the air for various population groups in Ahmedabad. *Atmosphere Environment*. 16(4):867–70.

Agrawal, A., Sharma a, Roychowdhury A. 1996: *Slow Murder: The Deadly Story of Vehicular Pollution in India*. New Delhi: Central Science Environment.

Almin, L. Schorr 1963: *Slums and social insecurity*, Nelson publications.

Alauddin, M. 1986: *"Maternal Mortality in rural Bangladesh: The tangail District"*. Studies in Family Planning.

Ambarasu, K, Bhaskaran. R, Ferozekhan. M, and Selvaraj. S, Deparment of Geology, National Collage Tiruchirapalli, India, 2004: *A Study of the Water Pollution of Kayalpattinam Area,* Tuticorin, Tamil Nadu, Journal of Industriel pollution control Vol, 20(1), 2004.

Anthony, A. D'Souza Alfred Souza (1972): *Population growth and human development*, Indian social institute, New Delhi.

Banta, Bob, 1993: *"Minority Community Grappling with Goals, Environmental Agenda"* Austin American-Statesman, Jan. 4.

Baljeets Kapoor, Byankteshnarayan and Mehrotra, 1999: *Defluoridation of Drinking Water Using Low Cost Absorbent.* Indian Journal of Environmental Health, Vol, 41, No, 1, P.53-58 (January 1999).

Berry, Brian J. L. 1977: *The Social Burdens of Environmental Pollution*: A Comparative study of Metropolitan data Source. Cambridge, Massachusetts: Ballinger.

Bhattacharjree, P.J. 1983: "*Role of internal migration in Karnataka's development*" published in Vastsala Narain and Prakasam C.P, Population policy perspectives in developing countries Himalaya Publishing house, Bombay.

Bibhu Prasad Tripathy, 2004: 'Public litigation' Environment support Group CEERA (ESG website)

Bridgeland, William M., and Andrew J. Sofranko, 1975: "*Community Structure and Issue Specific Influences; Community Mobilisation Over Environmental Quality,*" Urban Affairs Quarterly.

Bombay's survival kit, (2001): Poverty, Environment and disease in Bombay, E-Mail: Healthlibrary.com/reading/war/chap// .htm.

Buttel, Frederick, and William L. Flinn, 1978: "*Social Class and Mass Environmental Beliefs: A Reconsideration.*" *Environmental Behaviour.*

Buch, M.N. 1993: Environmental Consciousness and Urban Planning – TRACTS FOR THE TIMES / 2, Orient Longman limited.

Central Pollution Control Board, 1993, 94, 95: *Pollution Statistics* New Delhi: Central Pollution Control Board.

Chakrabarthi, T, 1993: *Legality of Hazardous Waste Management in India,* Journal of Indian Association for Environmental Management. Vol, 20, P, 1-3, 1993.

Chakravarti, S. 1998: Deals on wheels *India Today,* Jan. 19.

Cheney, Jim, 1987: "*Ecofeminism and Deep Ecology*" Environmental ethics, 9(2), Summer.

Chhatwal, G.R. 1993: "*Encyclopedia of Environmental pollution and its Control.* Anmol publications, New Delhi.

David, L. Morgan, 1988: *Portland State University, focus Groups as Qualitative Research, Qualitative Research Method volume-16,* Sage publications, the International professional publishers New bury part London, New Delhi.

David, R. Hunter, the slums: Challenge and response London, clothier Mc Millan Ltd.

Dankelman, Irene and Joan Davidson, 1988: *Women and the Environment in the third world*: Alliance for the future. London. Earth scan.

Department of Community Medicine Kempegowda Institute of medical sciences Jan-June-1998, Bangalore. India population project- VIII Bangalore, Indian journal of community Health, vol. 4

Devid, A.R. and Devadas pillai1972, cited in D.N.Dhanagere, 1998: Themes and perspectives in Indian Sociology, Rawat Publication, Jaipur, pp 59-60.

Development support and research division (1996): *Sector strategy paper on health Action AID*. 3. Rest house road Bangalore.

Department of Family Welfare, Ministry of Health and Family Welfare Govt. of India Reports, (Oct 1997): *Reproductive and child health programme schemes for implementation department.*

Devall, Bill 1992: *"Deep Ecology and Radical Environmentalism."* In Riley E. Dunlap and Angela G. Mertig. Eds. *American Environmentalism: The U.S. Environmental Movements* 1970-1990. new Yark: Taylor and Francis,

Dhadave, M.S. 1988, Sociology of slum, Archives Books, New Delhi-55

D'Souza, V.S " Slums and Social structure" Urban and Rural Planning Thought, 8(1-2)pp 70-74.

Dr. K.N. Venkatarayappa (1072): *SLUMS. [A STUDY IN URBAN PROBLEM.]* Sterling publishers. (p) LTD. New Delhi. pp. 3,4,5,6.

Dr. Ashok Sahni (1988): *Health of the metro polis Bangalore*: Indian Society of Health Administrators (ISHA).

Dr. Y. Narayana Chetty 2004: *DYNAMICS OF TRADE UNIONISM INDIA*, Anmol Publication PVT. LTD.

Dr. Y. Narayana Chetty, *Trade Union and Environment Consciousness - An Exploratory Sociological Analysis* - Paper presented at National Seminar on Environmental Knowledge and practices in India, organised by the Dept. of Sociology, Shivaji University Kolhapur. March 1998.

Dunlap, Riley E. 1975: *"The Socioeconomic Basis of the Environmental Movement: Old Data New Data, and Implications for the Movement's Future."* Paper presented at the annual meeting of the American Sociological Association. San Francisco, August 1975.

Eckersley, Robyn, 1992: *Environmentalism and Political Theory,* London: UCL Press.

Egbert Tellegen and Maarten Wolsink, University of Amsterdam, Netherlands 1994: *Society - Its Environment,* Gordon and Breach Science Publishers.

Egbert Tellegen and Martin Wolsink, 1994: Society and Its Environment. An Introduction University of Amsterdam, the Netherlands. pp. 6-21 and 81-90

Family Planning Association of India (Oct-1997): Planned Parenthood-3,Vol.5 No. 4

Ferris BG Jr, -Speizer FE, -Spengler JD, -1979: Effects of sulfur oxides and respirable particles on human health: methodology and demography of populations in study. *Am. Rev. Respiratory Disorders.* 120:76779

Francis Abraham, John Henry Morgan, *Social thought- From Comte to Sorokin,* Mac Millan India press Madras.

Frieden, Bernard J. 1979: *The Environmental Frotection Hustle.* Cambridge, M.A: The MIT Press.

Gamble, JF, -Lewis RJ. -1996: Health and Respirable Particulate (PM_{10}) Air Pollution: A Causal or Statistical Association? *Environmental Health Perspective.* 104:83850.

Gedicks, et. al. 1993: *The New Resource Wars: Native and Environmental Struggle against Multinational Corporations.* Boston: South End Press.

Ghosh, B.N. (2003), *Scientific Method and social Research,* New Delhi. Sterling publisher's private limited.

Gopeshnath Khanna, *Global Environmental crisis and management,* Ashish publishing house, New Delhi.

Government of India (1995), *Five Year Plans and Volumes,* Government Press.

Govt. of India (1991), *1991 Census Reports*, New Delhi, Govt. press.

Govt. of India 1996. Annual Report, 1995-1996: New Delhi: Ministry Of Power, Government of India.

Govt. of Karnataka *2001 Census*, Bangalore. Govt. press.

Hans Raj 2002: *Theory and practice in social research*, SURJEET PUBLICATIONS, New Delhi.

Indira Munshi, 2000: Faculty of the department of sociology, University of Mumbai: 'Environment' in Sociological Theory, SOCIOLOGICAL BULLETIN, 49(2), September 2000. pp. 258-262,

Indian conference of social work (1958), *Report on the seminar of slum clearance*, Bombay. Report.

International Standard Organisation. 1992: >*Air qualityparticle size fraction definitions for health-related sampling. Technical Report. ISO/TR/7708-1983 (E)*. Geneva: ISO

Iyengar, S. Keshava, and Aijer, C.P. Ramaswamy, Hydrabad, 1986: Decan India; *A Report on the Socio- economic and Health Survey of Street Baggers in Hyderabad- Secundrabad city areas: A Report.* Indian Institute of Economics Hyderabad.

Iyengar, S. Keshva, 1959: A *survey of hut dwellers in Hyderabad city.* Report. Indian Institute of Economics

Jadav, H.V. 1995: *"Environmental Pollution"*. Himalaya Publication House.

Jain, P.K, Piush Gupta, and Rajarishi Sinha, 1994: *Water Quality Modeling of a City Water Distribution System*, Indian Journal of Environmental Health, Vol. 36, No, 4, 258-262(October 1994).

Jean, M. Converse, 1986: University of Michigan Stanley presse-National science foundation. SURVEY QUESTIONS *handcrafting the Standardis*ed *Questionnaire*, Sage publications. The International professional publishers New Bury park London, New Delhi.

Jha, U.C. 2004: "Environmental Issues and SAARC", Economic and political weekly April 24, 2004.

Jonathan, H. Turner 2001: *The structure of sociological theory*, Rawat Publications Jaipur.

John, W. Creswell, *Qualitative enquiry and research design choosing among five traditions,* Sage, professional Publisher, Thousand Oaks, London, New Delhi.

Kamat, SR. -1984: *Bombay Air Pollution Health Study.* Bombay: Municipal. Corporation. Greater Bombay.

Kamat, SR, -Mahashur AA. -1997: *Air pollution: slow poisoning.* In *The Hindu Survey of the Environment* Madras: Hindu Press

Koteswara, Rao T. Director, Special Monitoring Cell Planning Department, 2000: Environmental statistics on human settlements through large scale socio-Economic sample survey in India.

Krishnan, M. 1994: Regional Cancer Centre, Thiruvananthapuram, Kerala, India: 'Environmental Issues' Journal of Environmental resources: Vol. 2: Nos.1-4: 1994: pp, 14-15.

Krishna Swamy O.R. 2001: *Methodology of research in social science* Mumbai. Himalaya Publishing house.

Kwitko, Ludmilla. 1994: *"Gender and Household Communities in Asia."* Paper presented at the Annual American Sociological Association Meet. Los Angeles, California: August 8, 1994.

Kudesia, V.P. 1980: Air Pollution Pragathi publication, Meerut, India.

Liz Creel (2002): Children's Environmental Health: Risks and Remedies, POPULATION REFERENCE BUREAU.

Lookman, AA, -Rubin ES. -1998: *Barriers to adopting least-cost particulate control strategies for Indian power plants. Energy Policy* 26(14):105363

Mathur, R.N 1986: *Population Analysis and studies,* CHUGH publications Alahabad India.

Mehra, A, Farago ME, -Banerjee DK. -1998: Impact of fly ash from coal-fired power stations in Delhi, with particular reference to metal contamination. *Environment Monitoring Assessment* 50 (1):1535

Milliam, Reidhead, P. Shuchi Gupta, Deepti Joshi. (1996): State of Indian's Environment A qualitative Analysis, Tata Energy Research Institute, Institute Delhi.

Mishra, V., Retherford RD, -Smith KR. -1997: *Effects of Cooking Smoke on Prevalence of Tuberculosis in India. East-West Centre Working Paper Population Series, No. 92.* East-West Centre, Honolulu, Hawaii

Mostardi, RA, -Leonard D. -1974: Air pollution and cardiopulmonary function. *Arch. Environ. Health* 29:32528

Morrison, Denton E., Kennath E. Hornback, and W.Keith Warner.1972: *"The Environmental Movement: Some Preliminary Observations and Predictions."* In William R. Burch. Neil H. Cheek, and Lee Taylor, eds. Social Behaviour, Natural Resources, and the Environment. New York: Harper and Row.

Nair, P.K.K. 1993: Emeritus Scientist CSIR (Council of Scientific and Industrial Research) Environmental Resources Research Centre Thiruvananthapuram, Kerala: *People's Participation In Environmental Movement, Journal of environmental Resources:* Vol. 1 : 1-2, 1993, pp1-3.

Parental Control, Delayed marriage and population policies (Reports) 1965: World Population Conference, Belgrade.

Paramesha Naik.D Ushamalani, Somashekar R.K.2004: Environmental Pollution Control Journal (A bi-monthly journal dedicated to environmental pollution, its causes & remedies etc., Vol.8, No.1 November – December 2004.

Pragya Sharma, Dr. Amareet Kaur 1999: *Removal of a basic dye from aqueous solution using various types of low cost adsorbents,* Environmental Pollution Control Journal, Jan-Feb, G.J. University Hisar, Dr. Dilip Kumar Markendsy from CPCB, New Delhi 1999.

Prasad, P.M, January 17, 2004: (Much of the material has been drawn from) article published in special article, Environmental Protection: The role of Liability System in India, By, Economic and Political Weekly, PP. 257-259

Praveen, Visaria and Leel Visaria (1981): *Indian population Scence after 1981 censes,* Sameeksha Trust publication, journal: Economic and political weekly, special number.Nov-1981.

Population council, Population briefs. (sep-2000): Urban states slum residence and adverse health consequences linked in keenya.

Power, R, 2002: *Research Methods- The application of Qualitative Research methods to the study of sexually transmitted Infections:* London UK 18 February-2002.

Rajeev Koshal (1996): *Population Growth and Family welfare Programme in India,* APH Publication Corporation. New Delhi.

Rekha Ghosh, Chatterjee 2004: Environmental Geology, Geo-ecosystem Protection in Mining Area, Capital Publishing company New Delhi.

Reports 1997: *White Paper on Pollution in Delhi with an Action Plan.* New Delhi: Ministry of Environment. Government of India.

Riley, E. Dunlap and Angela G. Mertig, eds.1992: *Mobilising the African-American Community for Social Change. American Environmentalism: The U.S. Environmental Movement 1970-1990.* Philadelphia: Taylor-Francis.

Robson, B.T. 1971: Urban Analysis-A study of city with reference to sundarlana structure Introductory Industrial Sociology. Cambridge University, Cambridge University press,

Rodda, Annabel. 1991: *Women and the Environment*. London: Sed Books.

Sharma, R.N, R.K. Sharma.1999: *Introductory Industrial sociology* Bombay, Media promoters and publishers Pvt. Ltd.

Shah, J, -Nagpal T,- eds. 1997: *Urban Air Quality Management Strategy in Asia (URBAIR). Greater Mumbai Reports. World Bank Tech. Pap. No. 381,* World Bank, Washington, DC

Shah, N, Ramankutty V, -Premila PG, -Sathy N. -1994: Risk factors for severe pneumonia in children in south Kerala: a hospital-based case-control study. *J. Trop. Pediatr.* 40(4):2016

Shiva, Vandana. 1989: Staying Alive: *Women, Ecology and Development*. London: Sed Books.

Sir Claus Moser, Director, Central Statistical Office, and Kalton.G Leverhulme Professor of Social Statistics University of Southampton1971: Survay of Methods in Social Investigation. Heinemann Educational Books, LONDON.

Singh, R.L. (1964): An Urban survey" National Geological Society of India Varanasi.

Smith, KR. 1993: Fuel combustion, air pollution exposure, and health: the situation in developing countries. Annu. Rev. Energy Environ. 18:52966

Smith, KR. 1999: *The national burden of disease from indoor air pollution in India.*Paper Presented at Indoor Air '99, Edinburgh, UK

Smith, KR, Liu Y. 1994: *Indoor air pollution in developing countries in The Epidemiology of Lung Cancer,* ed. J Samet, pp. 15184. New York: Marcel Dekker

Smt. Swati Ramanathan(2003): *Participatory planning: A, Citizen's Hand Book,* Ramanathan Foundation Bangalore.

Srinivas, M.N. M.S.A. Rao. A.M. Shah. (1974): *A survey of research in social Anthropology,* Manmohan.S. Bhatkak. At popular Book Depot printing division. Sponsor by: Indian Council of Social Science Research.

Suma, Tekur Deccan Herald 26th January, 2004: Toxics Link. 2003, scrapping the hi-tech myth - Computer waste in India, 2002.

Sunil kumar, Snigeo Shikura, Hideki Harada, (2003): *Living Environment and Health of urban poor,* journal: Economic and political weekly, Vol:6 No.Aug-2003. Samiksha Trust publication.

Tata Energy Research Institute. (Reports)1993: *Impact of Road Transportation on Energy and EnvironmentAn Analysis of Metropolitan Cities of India.* New Delhi: TERI (TATA ENERGY RESEARCH INSTITUTE)

Thomas, Caroline, 1992: *The Environment in International Relations.* London: Royal Institute of International Affairs.

Tripathi, A. 1994: Airborne lead pollution in the city of Varanasi, India. *Atmosphere Environment* 28:231723

Tripathi, R.S. and R.P. Thivari: *Population Growth and Development in India* ASIA PUBLISHING HOUSE.

Tripathi, RM, -Khandekar RN, -Raghunath R, -Mishra UC. -1989: Short communication: assessment of atmospheric pollution from toxic heavy metals in two cities in India. *Atmosphere Environment* 23:87983.

US Environmental Protection Agency. 1973: *Mobile Source Emission Standards Summary.* Washington, DC: US EPA. 2nd edition.

US Environmental Protection Agency. 1982: *Review of the National Ambient Air Quality Standard for Particulate Matter: Assessment of Scientific and Technical Information*. Research Triangle Park, NC: US EPA

US Environmental Protection Agency. 1985: *Compilation of Air Pollutant Emission Factors. EPA Manual AP-42, Suppl. A.* Research Triangle Park, NC: US EPA. 4th ed.

Wang, XD, -Smith KR. -1999: Secondary benefits of greenhouse gas control: health impacts in China. *Environ. Sci. Technol.* 33(18):305661

Weston, Joe, 1986: *"The Greens. 'Nature', and The Social Env8ironment." In Joe Weston, ed. Red and Green: A New Politics of the Environment.* London and Wolfeboro, NH: Pluto press.

WHO, 1992: *Programme for Control of Acute Respiratory Infections. WHO/ARI/92.22.* Geneva: WHO

Workplace Atmospheres, 1992: Size Fraction Definitions for Measurement of Airborne Particles in the Workplace. CEN Stand. EN 481. CEN

WHO, 1993: *Assessment of Sources of Air, Water, and Land Pollution. A Guide to Rapid Source Inventory Techniques and Their Use in Formulating Environmental Control Strategies. Part 1. Rapid Inventory Techniques in Environmental Pollution. WHO/PEP/GETNET/93.1-A.* Geneva: WHO

WHO, 1997: *Tobacco or Health: A Global Status Report*. Geneva: WHO

WHO/UN Environmental Programme. 1992: *Urban Air Pollution in Mega-cities of the World*. Oxford: Blackwell.

World Research Institute 1998-99: *Health and Environment, Improving through Environment Action taking the problems of poverty environment and health.*

18/01/2002, Prajavani.

09/01/2002, Samyuktha Karnataka.

2/05/2002, Times of India.

3/05/2002. Times of India.

05/01/2002, Vijay Karnataka.

13/03/2002, Vijay Karnataka.

15/03/2002, Vijay Karnataka.

26/03/2000, Vijay Karnataka.

Index

F

G

H

I

J

K

L

M

N

P

R

S